Interactive Group Learning

Strategies for Nurse Educators

Second Edition

Deborah Ulrich, PhD, RN, has been a nurse educator for the past 30 years in diverse educational settings. She has influenced nursing education through journal articles, books, and national presentations focusing on innovative teaching strategies. Debbie received her B.S.N. from The Ohio State University, her Masters from Ball State University in Muncie, Indiana, and her Doctorate from The Ohio State University. Presently, she is a professor of nursing at Miami University in Ohio and teaches in the baccalaureate nursing program.

Kellie Glendon, MSN, RNC, is an experienced nurse educator, author, and national speaker on innovative teaching in nursing curricula. She received her B.S.N. from The College of Mt. St. Joseph on the Ohio and her Masters from the University of Cincinnati, Cincinnati, Ohio. Kellie has received certification in obstetrics. Presently she is an associate professor of nursing at Miami University and has been teaching students in the Associate Degree Nursing Program for the past 15 years. She was awarded the Excellence in Teaching Award by the Greater Cincinnati Consortium of Colleges and Universities in 1998.

Since Debbie and Kellie began working together they have published numerous journal articles on innovative teaching and learning, co-authored two books, *Interactive Group Learning: Strategies for Nurse Educators* and *Unfolding Case Studies: Experiencing the Realities of Clinical Nursing Practice* (Springer, 1999), spoken at over 50 national nurse educator conferences, and consulted with numerous schools of nursing on creative and interactive teaching modalities. As of January 2004 they are co-authoring the bimonthly column, "Dear Florence," in *Nurse Educator*.

Interactive Group Learning

Strategies for Nurse Educators

Second Edition

Deborah L. Ulrich, PhD, RN
Kellie J. Glendon, MSN, RN, C

 Springer Publishing Company

Springer Publishing Company, Inc.
11 West 42nd Street, 15th Floor
New York, NY 10036-8002

Acquisitions Editor: Ruth Chasek
Production Editor: Jeanne W. Libby
Cover design by Joanne Honigman

05 06 07 08 09 / 5 4 3 2 1

Library of Congress Cataloging-in-Publication Data

Ulrich, Deborah L.
  Interactive group learning : strategies for nurse educators / Deborah L. Ulrich, Kellie J. Glendon. — 2nd ed.
      p. ; cm.
  Includes bibliographical references and index.
  ISBN 0-8261-3105-0
  1. Nursing—Study and teaching (Continuing education) 2. Group work in education. 3. Active learning.
  [DNLM: 1. Education, Nursing—methods. 2. Group Structure. 3. Learning.] I. Glendon, Kellie J. II. Title.
  RT76.U46 2005
  610.73'071'1—dc22   2005004764

Printed in the United States of America by Sheridan Books.

Contents

Preface

We initially decided to write the first edition of this book because, as graduates of Miami University's Teaching Scholars Program, we had experienced the essence of teaching and learning and realized that teaching was more than telling. After experimenting with group-learning strategies we found that our students were capable of much more than we were giving them credit for. They began to ask thought-provoking questions and then found the answers themselves, as we facilitated the group process. We then began to publish our experiences and speak about them at national conferences. Seeing the interest and enthusiasm of other nurse educators across the country, we felt compelled to share our insights and successes with them so that they could also see their students develop intellectually. Writing the second edition of the book seems a natural progression. We have grown in our insights, as well as in the scope of the creative strategies we use on a daily basis. We have networked extensively with other educators who have used our strategies, evaluated their effectiveness, and encouraged us to continue developing innovative group learning techniques that help us educate professional nurses for the twenty-first century. Our hope is that by sharing our ideas through this book, nursing faculty everywhere will be motivated to continue the quest for more and better ways to help students learn!

DEBORAH ULRICH
KELLIE GLENDON

Acknowledgments

We wish to thank our students at Miami University who have helped us to learn how to teach more effectively and how to empower them to become active lifelong learners. We wish to thank Miami University's Alumni Teaching Scholars Program for bringing us together as colleagues and scholars interested in finding a better way to teach our students.

We wish to thank faculty across the country who have attended our workshops, read our articles, and encouraged us to continue to share interactive teaching strategies with the nurse educator community.

We wish to thank Dr. Suzanne P. Smith, editor of *Nurse Educator*, for publishing our creative ideas and allowing us to share our expertise with faculty across the country through the bimonthly column "Dear Florence."

Introduction

It is certainly not current news that educators are beginning to look critically at the teaching learning process, yet it has been only in the last several years that nursing has begun to implement these new ideas. As veteran nurse educators, we have experimented with innovative and creative teaching strategies since the early 1990s, and we feel that we have gained much insight into the process of learning. We have discovered that a central tenet of effective learning is active involvement. Students who are actively involved in the learning process learn not only essential content more effectively, but also the crucial skills of communicating and interacting with others. More than ever before, nurses are expected to think on their feet and efficiently apply their knowledge in situations with clients who are more acutely ill, are experiencing complex health problems, or present with a complicated and often dysfunctional family history. Nurses must be able to collaborate with other health care professionals, refer their clients to resources available in the community, as well as serve as an advocate for their clients and their families. These responsibilities require nurses to learn more than just necessary medical knowledge. It is essential for nurses to know how to work effectively with others, think critically, and communicate in speaking, writing, and interacting with others to benefit their clients. We have found that interactive group learning challenges students to meet these new learning essentials. This book is designed to help nurse educators or graduate students learning the art of teaching to implement this new group learning model in the undergraduate classroom and change the traditional education paradigm. It could also be used by staff educators for the continuing education of practicing nurses. These experienced nurses often bring a wealth of knowledge regarding real-life situations that augment the learning for the entire group.

This book is divided into six chapters that present clear and practical ways to implement interactive group learning methods. Examples can be quickly integrated into your existing teaching plan and will add the dimension of critical thinking and problem solving abilities, skills crucial for work in today's fast-changing health care environment.

Chapter 1 describes the shift in thinking about education from the traditional "Instruction Paradigm" to the new "Learning Paradigm." It details the advantages of this new paradigm and challenges you, the educator, to examine your curriculum and adapt your teaching methods to promote critical thinking and experiential learning through cooperative group techniques.

Chapter 2 presents our Comprehensive Group Learning Model designed to help you visualize the overall design of group learning through individual preparation, group interaction and sharing, and individual reflection. It explains the change in the teacher's role from one of information giver to one of facilitator and consultant, as well as the change of student role from one of passive recipient of knowledge to one of active participant in the learning process. This model allows you to plan a total class experience that requires not only group activities, but builds in individual accountability and preparation. This chapter also discusses the intricacies and challenges of group learning. Group dynamics, peer and group evaluations are detailed. Problems frequently faced by faculty when managing student groups are discussed at length.

Chapter 3 discusses a multitude of cooperative learning strategies that can be used individually or in combination to cover the entire class content or as a break from traditional lecture. Each strategy is explained in enough detail to allow you, the teacher, to read it and immediately implement it in the classroom as a part of your already prepared lecture or class discussion. It also shows you how to combine a multitude of these cooperative strategies to teach an entire class, covering all of the content you need to teach. All of the strategies described stimulate group interaction and problem solving.

Chapter 4 discusses the "Unfolding Case" and the "Unfolding Family Case" models. These examples show you how these models can be implemented in a nursing classroom, illustrating the total application of the "Comprehensive Group Learning Model."

Chapter 5 introduces you to ways to involve students holistically through their senses. These strategies will help you enhance students' critical thinking abilities and allow them the experience of working with others at the same time. The chapter discusses such activities as drawings, photographs, concept mapping, fishbone, games, and numerous other holistic strategies.

Chapter 6 shows you how to use writing to increase learning and help students reflect on classroom content, readings, professional issues, and their own thinking. It discusses ways to use both group writing and individual writing assignments to increase insight and encourage perspective taking on the part of our students. This chapter enumerates the benefits of teaching students how to use writing as a method of communicating, critiquing others in a thoughtful and methodical way, and explaining their own thinking, to name a few.

It is our hope that this handbook of interactive group learning strategies will assist you as you try to incorporate new ideas about teaching and learning into your classroom, as well as augment your existing repertoire of teaching strategies. We have found these strategies effective with all content common to general undergraduate nursing curricula, and think almost any material could be covered using these methods. We hope to stimulate you through this book to try new things by using our ideas, adapting our strategies to fit your own needs, or creating your own group learning techniques. Experiment! Have fun and share your newfound enthusiasm with others—it's contagious and we all need to be revitalized as we continue to take on the important task of educating nurses for the next century.

Chapter 1

Changing Classroom Dynamics for Learning Communities

T here has been a shift in thinking over the years about the educational process among faculty in higher education. Historically, educators provided instruction, were the center of knowledge, and imparted their expertise to students in the form of a formal lecture. Barr and Tagg (1995, p. 13) coined this traditional teaching–learning structure the "Instruction Paradigm." It is based on the ideas of John Locke (1693) who felt that a student's mind was a blank slate ("tabula rasa") and that a teacher's job was to fill that slate. He believed that a pupil was a modable entity, a person who could be improved by a good education and corrupted by a bad one. Hence, the idea of an active teacher and a passive student evolved and remained the norm for centuries. The new structure of teaching–learning is referred to as the "Learning Paradigm" and emphasizes learning rather than teaching. It involves students actively constructing their own knowledge, whereas the teacher's job changes to one of manipulating the environment to allow active student *discovery* of knowledge (see Table 1.1). This philosophical shift in emphasis from teaching to learning demands that educators examine their curricula and change their teaching methodologies to meet the emphasis on critical thinking and problem solving.

No longer can faculty pour information into students and expect that this alone will prepare them for the needs of tomor-

TABLE 1.1   Comparison of Characteristics of the Old Instructional Paradigm Versus the New Learning Paradigm

Instructional Paradigm	Learning Paradigm
Teacher is the expert and center of knowledge	Teacher is the facilitator of learning
Individual and competitive learning	Group, cooperative, and collaborative learning
Students are passive in the learning process	Students are actively involved in the learning process
Teaching is "telling" and giving knowledge	Teaching is structuring the environment so that students "discover" knowledge
Students listen, record, memorize, and regurgitate information	Students apply knowledge, think critically, communicate effectively, and reflect on their own learning

row's world (see Figure 1.1). Educators are beginning to evaluate the actual merits of this methodology of feeding students volumes of information much like a mother bird feeding her young. What could they expect to receive but the same information regurgitated back to them on an examination? Is this learning, or is it merely testing one's short-term memory? These are the questions that are now being contemplated by educators worldwide as they look more deeply at the way we have traditionally viewed the teaching–learning process.

Although students do need to know certain facts before they can apply and critically think about them, memorization should not be the end of the learning process but the starting point. Bombarding students with new facts and information in lecture form and expecting them to apply the information in a clinical situation, sometimes the very next day, only overwhelms them (see Figure 1.2). They need time and help in learning to apply these essential facts after learning them cognitively. Learning experts report that students retain only 20% of what they hear in a lecture and even less of what they read on their own (Ekwall, 1976). In

FIGURE 1.1   Professor "pouring" knowledge into the student.

fact, Silberman (1996) notes that teachers speak 100 to 200 words per minute, but even a student who is concentrating can hear only 50 to 100 words per minute. However, more information is learned and retained when students are involved in the educational process and actually participate in the process (Dale, 1969). It appears that in using traditional methods, educators tend to ignore the processing of information and instead focus on presenting material. It is clear that students retain more when they are active participants in processing the information rather than passive recipients of the knowledge (Kuhn, 2000; McKeachie, 1978). We also know that employers want to hire students who think critically, interact skillfully with others, and reflect on their own learning to improve themselves continuously. It is this kind of individual that will be successful now and in the future, long after the facts they

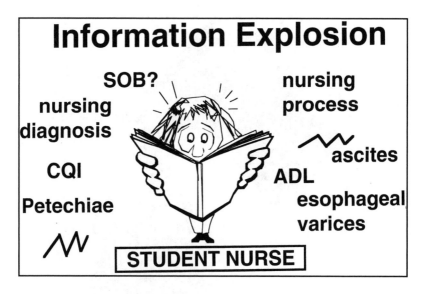

FIGURE 1.2   **Bombarding students with information.**

learned are outdated. So it is apparent that the outcomes faculty members need to produce in their students are the ability to think critically, problem solve, and remember and apply pertinent information—skills that will serve them well in life as well as in the role of a professional nurse.

CRITICAL THINKING AND REFLECTION

Critical thinking and reflection are two skills that we, as educators, need to require of our students. It is an evolving concept and not easily defined. The roots of critical thinking can be traced to Socrates 2500 years ago with his method of probing questioning to help people rationally justify their claims to knowledge. Plato and Aristotle followed his ideas and emphasized that things are often different than they appear, and we must train our minds to look beyond the surface. In time, other great thinkers such as Francis Bacon, René Descartes, Robert Boyle, and Sir Isaac Newton embraced the idea of using systematic critical thinking and the need for clarity and precision in thinking. A unifying thread in early thinkers was their ability to question commonly held knowledge and continually reflect on unexplained problems of the times. Every part of thinking was doubted, questioned, and tested. This led to the abandonment of irrational views in favor of ideas based on sound reasoning.

Thinking critically involves several skills that are best integrated through experiences (see Figure 1.3). In investigating the literature related to critical thinking we find substantial information, all defining, characterizing, and interpreting the term *critical thinking* in different but congruent ways. Watson and Glaser (1964) describe it as a combination of abilities needed to define problems, recognize assumptions, formulate and select hypotheses, draw conclusions, and judge validity of inferences. Ennis (1989) defines it as reasonable and reflective thinking, focused on deciding what to believe or what to do. Paul (1992) sees it as a process of self-disciplined and self-directed rational thinking that verifies what

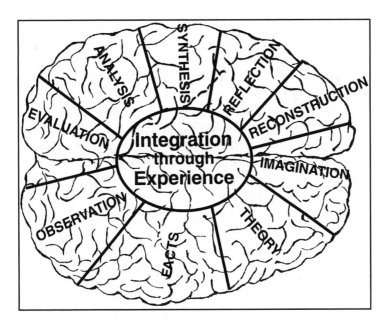

FIGURE 1.3   Critical thinking integrated through experience.

we know and clarifies what we don't know. Facione, Facione, and Sanchez (1994) characterize it as purposeful and self-regulatory judgments that result in interpretation, analysis, inference, evaluation, and explanation. Alfaro-LeFevre (1994) proposed that critical thinking was careful, deliberate, and goal directed. Bandman and Bandman (1995) state that critical thinking in nursing involves rational examination of ideas, inferences, assumptions, principles, arguments, conclusions, issues, statements, beliefs, and actions. Brookfield (1989) discovered that this concept has been likened to the development of logical reasoning, the use and testing of meaning, the application of reflective judgment, and the justification of beliefs. He sums it up best when he notes that critical thinking incorporates three closely related concepts: *emancipatory learning, dialectical thinking,* and *reflective learning* (Brookfield, 1989, p. 12). *Emancipatory learning* refers to individuals being free from societal constraints that force them to conform to learning in only traditional styles where the professor is the center of knowledge. It requires students to feel free to brainstorm, think critically, and question authority without the fear of being "put down." *Dialectical thinking* assumes that change is a reality and, hence, promotes a constant process to discover truth. In other words, students need to be taught that the only reality in life is change and that change is good and necessary for growth. This type of learning questions the norm and uses divergent thinking as a stimulus to further intellectual development. The *reflective* component of critical thinking involves looking at the justification for our beliefs and ideas or, more specifically, at the rationale for our actions. Why do I believe that, or what led me to this conclusion? If one is to accept something as truth, one must analyze the thought processes that led to acceptance of that fact.

Critical thinking in nursing similarly involves learning facts and applying them to common nursing situations. This involves examining multiple perspectives, analyzing and questioning assumptions, and interpreting information. Higher level thinking skills allow nurses to synthesize or reconstruct new concepts from data already known, as well as evaluate or judge the effectiveness of reasoned conclusions and their potential consequences. As practitioners, nurses will be faced with many decisions, some even life and death situations. Although there are certain facts nurses need to know to practice their profession safely, applying these facts to actual situations using the skill of critical thinking will enable them to solve problems effectively.

Faculty should feel obligated to teach students how to think and problem solve, not just teach reams of information. That conclusion implies that there is a way to teach someone to think critically, and it is this ability that is necessary for faculty members to use as they go about their business of educating practitioners for the twenty-first century. This can be accomplished by devising teaching strategies that require critical thinking abilities, such as identifying similarities and differences, comparing multiple perspectives, interpreting and using theory, clarifying and analyzing issues, making interdisciplinary connections, and generating and assessing solutions (see Table 1.2). These can be actualized by involving students in group activities that require problem solving.

One way faculty can stimulate students' thinking through these activities is to include pertinent focused questions (Glendon & Ulrich, 1997) that direct their learning and help them concentrate on the most essential information and skills (see Table 1.3). These questions serve as a "map" to students as they learn to use these thinking skills and practice applying them to the problems of nursing. However, it is imperative that faculty understand that just asking questions blindly will not necessarily result in critical thinking. Students need to learn basic facts and terms before critical thinking skills can be developed (Meyers, 1991). According to Paul and Elder (2001), there are three categories of questions: (1) questions with one right answer (facts), (2) questions that call for answers that are sheer opinion or preference, and (3) questions that require reasoned judgment. The first kind of question is the type we want to ask when students are mastering basic terms, concepts, and methodologies. The second type of question is valuable in helping students develop values and beliefs that help them discern where their strengths and interests lie. It is the third kind of question, though, that encourages critical thinking and can be rationally evaluated using universal intellectual standards such as clarity, depth, consistency, relevance, and so forth. We as faculty must teach students that they cannot use opinions for questions

TABLE 1.2   Selection of Critical Thinking Abilities

Identification and recognition abilities
  Identifying and recognizing elements of reasoning
  Uncovering significant similarities and differences
  Recognizing contradictions, inconsistencies, and double standards

Comprehension abilities: comparing and clarifying
  Uncovering significant similarities and differences
  Refining generalizations and avoiding oversimplifications
  Clarifying and analyzing issues, conclusions, or beliefs
  Clarifying and analyzing the meanings of words or phrases
  Developing criteria for evaluation: clarifying values and standards
  Comparing and contrasting ideals with actual practice
  Reasoning dialogically: comparing perspectives, interpretations, or theories

Application abilities
  Comparing analogous situations: transferring insights to new contexts
  Clarifying and analyzing the meanings of words or phrases
  Analyzing and evaluating arguments, interpretations, beliefs, or theories
  Analyzing and evaluating actions or policies
  Rethinking your thinking: metacognition
  Exploring thoughts underlying feelings and feelings underlying thoughts

Synthesis abilities
  Reasoning dialogically: comparing perspectives, interpretations, or theories
  Comparing analogous situations: transferring insights to new contexts
  Making interdisciplinary connections
  Reasoning dialectically: evaluating perspectives, interpretations, or theories

Evaluation abilities
  Refining generalizations and avoiding oversimplifications
  Comparing and contrasting ideals with actual practice
  Designing and carrying out tests of concepts, theories, and hypotheses
  Analyzing and evaluating arguments, interpretations, beliefs, or theories
  Analyzing and evaluating actions or policies
  Rethinking your thinking: metacognition
  Exploring thoughts underlying feelings and feelings underlying thoughts
  Reasoning dialectically: evaluating perspectives, interpretations, or theories
  Evaluating the credibility of sources of information
  Generating and assessing solutions
  Questioning deeply: raising and pursuing root or significant questions

Abilities to create or generate
  Designing and carrying out tests of concepts, theories, and hypotheses
  Generating and assessing solutions
  Creating concepts, arguments, or theories

From Paul, R. (1993). *Critical thinking: How to prepare students for a rapidly changing world.* Santa Rosa, CA: Foundation for Critical Thinking. Reprinted by permission.

TABLE 1.3   Focused Questions

Factually Based
    What is the definition of an induced abortion?

Opinion Based
    What do you believe about women who seek and obtain abortions and why?

Reason Based
    What are the pros and cons of obtaining an abortion from the client's point
    of view?

that require reasoning, because in doing so, they are practicing pseudo-critical thinking. They must realize that they need to provide legitimate reasons and evidence in supporting their answers if they are truly thinking critically.

EXPERIENTIAL LEARNING

Experiential learning provides the link between critical thinking and student involvement. It is, in fact, the process we often use when teaching the skill of critical thinking. Dewey (1944) observed, as early as 1915, that learning occurs in society as a result of social interaction. He thought that formal education needed to be active and that students needed to be involved, or experience the knowledge firsthand, if they were to discover the "connections of things" (Dewey, 1944, p. 340). The Gestalt theorists Wertheimer and later Koffka, Kohler, and Lewin studied the relationship or link between experience (as defined by Dewey) and learning (Bigge, 1971). They determined that experiential learning helped students develop reflective thinking skills that, in turn, enabled them to transfer knowledge to new situations (Bigge, 1971). Many educators have used the principles of Dewey and the Gestalt theorists to develop teaching strategies, such as simulations, role play, and laboratory experiences. Frederick (1990) used stories, writing exercises, music, and dynamic visuals to "connect" the student's life experiences to the subject matter at hand. Tapping students holistically (i.e., physically, intellectually, emotionally, and spiritually) allows them to become more actively involved or connected to the learning experience. They, in fact, experience learning firsthand as they are forced to participate actively in the process. Experiential learning activities that tap the senses and the emotional and psychological facets of the student extend the effectiveness of the learning outcome produced.

COOPERATIVE LEARNING

Cooperative learning adds yet another dimension to Fredericks's ideas (1990): the social dimension, which binds students together to solve problems or learn specific content. It is the process by which students implement the teacher-planned activities. "Cooperative learning is an interactive teaching strategy that stimulates critical thinking, fosters a feeling of community within the group and promotes individual responsibility for learning through group process techniques" (Glendon & Ulrich, 1992a, p. 37). Students learn not only how to think and analyze but also how to work effectively in teams, learning outcomes useful in the work world.

Group processing through cooperative structures involves students working in groups of four to six members. Groups can be formed by random choices, self-selection, or teacher decisions. Working in heterogeneous groups gives students experiences in interacting with others who come from multiple perspectives, such as different cultures, achievement levels, learning styles, sex, and ages. Hence, deliberately formed groups that are heterogeneous seem to work best. Group work helps students develop crucial communication skills needed for building consensus, disagreeing with others with divergent ideas while maintaining respect for one another, encouraging and including others in discussion, and resolving conflict. In fact, cooperative learning stresses the development of social skills as well as cognitive ones.

Cooperative learning is not a new concept in education. In fact, much research has been done dealing with the effectiveness of these methods. Research has consistently shown that cooperative learning methods not only produce greater academic achievement than do traditional methods of instruction but also improve student self-esteem, promote positive attitudes about school, and encourage interaction between students of different types (Sharan, 1980; Slavin, 1980, 1983a, 1983b). Although, traditionally, most research has been conducted on the kindergarten through 12th-grade level, one early college-level nursing study found that African-American nursing students studying cooperatively achieved higher scores on state board examinations than a control group that studied independently (Frierson, 1986). In recent years, both interest in and research on cooperative learning have consistently increased in higher education and the same benefits as seen at younger educational levels have been found (Cooper & Mueck, 1990; Johnson, Johnson, & Smith, 1991; Qin, Johnson, & Johnson, 1995). In fact, research has shown that "cooperative efforts produce higher quality problem solving than do competitive efforts on a wide variety of problems that require different cognitive processes to solve" (Qin et al., 1995, p. 139). In summary, there seem to be four major benefits of cooperative learning: (1) increased student involvement, (2) enhancement of critical thinking, (3) improved communication, and (4) promotion of responsibility for learning.

Although the terms *group learning* and *cooperative learning* are often used synonymously, they have substantial differences. Cooperative learning has several characteristics that distinguish it from traditional small-group learning, group projects, or buzz groups (Cuseo, 1992). Cooperative-learning groups are intentionally formed to assure heterogeneity; they do not form by chance or student choice. Generally these groups meet regularly for an extended period of time and do not change every class period as small-group work groups may. This longevity promotes cohesiveness and a group bond. Efforts are aimed, through specific activities, to promote cooperation and interdependence among team members. In a cooperative learning classroom, four principles should be present: positive interdependence, individual accountability, equal participation of all group members, and simultaneous interaction of group members (Ledlow, 1999).

Communication and social interaction skills are stressed as groups interact, and specific exercises are included in the group work assignments to assure this focus. In cooperative learning groups, the instructor acts as a facilitator and consultant as the group processes its task, whereas in traditional group work the instructor leaves the students to go about their work with little structure.

Kagan (1989–1990) illustrates the point that all classroom instruction has a particular structure, even the "whole class question-and-answer" strategy, but the level of participation of each student—and, hence, learning—is in question in this and other traditional structures. For example, in this structure, the teacher calls on one student, and the student tries to answer correctly. With the "whole class question and answer," it is usually higher achieving students who have the most poise, confidence, and knowledge level that participate, whereas lower achievers with less self-esteem may sit and listen, or even tune out. Learning is more apt to be meaningful if all students take part in the group-learning structures. These structures designed by the authors and other cooperative-learning experts tend to multiply the learning potential in the classroom by assuring that more than a select few students are involved. Examples of these structures applied to nursing education and staff development are provided in detail throughout this book. In addition, there are several cooperative learning workbooks that are excellent references for college teachers wanting to change their teaching style to include group learning structures (Cooper et al., 1990; Goodsell, Maber, & Tinto, 1992; Johnson, Johnson, & Smith, 1991, 1998; Kagan, 1992; Millis & Cottell, 1998; Solomon, Davidson, & Solomon, 1993).

In summary, the new learning paradigm is here, and it is time for nurse educators to analyze its value and experiment with it in their own classrooms. Together we can improve the learning, skill, and potential of the professional nurses of tomorrow.

CHAPTER 2

The Comprehensive Group Learning Model and the Intricacies and Challenges of Group Interaction

It is readily apparent that to teach in this new learning paradigm, faculty members need to mesh the concepts of critical thinking, experiential learning, reflection, and cooperative learning in such a way as to accomplish the desired educational outcomes of producing students who can think, analyze, problem solve, communicate, and evaluate their own effectiveness to assure self-improvement. However, facts and knowledge cannot be forgotten as they are prerequisite to one's ability to analyze and problem solve. How can we, as faculty, assure that our students receive both? Figure 2.1 describes the use of a *Comprehensive Group-Learning Model* that does just that. Faculty can use it to design individual classes or even entire courses that meet the desired outcomes of learning facts as well as critical analyses.

In this model, the teacher's role changes to one of facilitator and consultant. The facilitator acts as a guide by creating an environment that is conducive to learning. It becomes the teacher's job to help students discover the material rather than outlining it for them. After the teacher sets up the experience, the students first prepare individually out of class through teacher-constructed study guides (see Table 2.1), worksheets, and other exercises that require them to attain essential factual information, and then, in groups, become active participants in solving the problem or

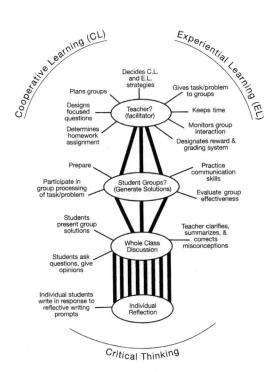

FIGURE 2.1   Comprehensive group learning model.

completing the task at hand. The problem often includes focused questions (see Table 1.3) that guide students to practice and apply the principles of critical thinking. These problem-based activities are processed through cooperative-learning strategies or structures that enhance or augment the level of participation of every student. Through teacher-planned activities, student groups generate solutions and share their results with the entire class. The facilitator (teacher) circulates in the room, keeping time, clarifying the task, and monitoring the groups' interactions. Students are encouraged by the facilitator to promote cohesiveness of their groups by practicing social relationship skills and communication techniques, such as active listening, paraphrasing, clarifying, brainstorming, and conflict resolution. The teacher than facilitates a total class interaction, promoting a higher level of discussion and analysis, which

TABLE 2.1   Example of a Study Guide for Cystic Fibrosis

Cystic Fibrosis (CF) (Wong, 1999, pp. 1518–1527)

1. What is the incidence of CF?
2. What culture is primarily affected?
3. Because this is a genetic, autosomal recessive disease, what is the chance of two people with the trait conceiving a child with CF?
4. What is the estimated life expectancy of children with CF?
5. What is the basic clinical feature of CF?
6. Describe how the functional patterns are affected by CF.

Activity Exercise
What respiratory assessments are common?
What treatments can the nurse perform to loosen secretions?
What common drugs are administered to reduce infectious processes?
Describe the teaching parents will need related to central lines, venous access ports for home care.
What other respiratory treatments will parents need to learn to manage?
How do hot weather and exercise influence children with CF?

Nutrition-Metabolic
Why do these children have poor weight gain and a thin, underdeveloped appearance?
What medications are used to enhance nutritional absorption?
What supplemental feedings are generally used at night?
Describe the teaching needed for parents/child related to nasogastric or nasojejunal tube feedings.
What contributes to the bleeding tendency in the child with advanced CF disease?
What disease leads to additional nutrition problems in a child with advanced disease?

Role Relationship
How can nurses support families experiencing CF?

Self-Perception
Explain how individuals are affected by this disease.
What is the effect of having CF on development, especially adolescence?
What interventions can nurses encourage to influence a positive self-concept?

Elimination
What assessment is critical in newborns to monitor for this problem early on?
What are the characteristics of stools?
Why is there an increased chance of bowel obstruction and prolapse of the rectum?

highlights the critical thinking component. Students are finally asked to reflect on their own learning experiences through a short writing exercise. This writing exercise provides closure to the discussion, adds a new component for thought, or encourages students to evaluate their own effectiveness. Table 2.2 lists some selected reflective writing prompts. Reflective writing provides an individual critical thinking moment and is essential to the overall goals of learning, helping students to improve themselves continuously by encouraging them to think about what they have learned and how it will personally affect them. It is an important element completing the Comprehensive Group-Learning Model.

IMPLEMENTING A GROUP LEARNING MODEL

It is obvious from the literature that the use of group-learning strategies that allow students to be active and involved in the learn-

TABLE 2.2   Reflective-Thinking and Writing Prompts for Writing Exercises

What are your beliefs about _____?

How have your beliefs about _____ been changed?

What is your interpretation of _____?

Write a reaction to _____ from the perspective of the nurse/patient/family.

Write a critique of your group's discussion.

List two ways in which your group could be more effective.

Describe one way to keep a group member from dominating the discussion.

Describe one way to help a shy group member to contribute to the discussion.

Summarize the essence of the argument for or against _____.

Write supporting statements of an argument that you truly do not support.

Write objectives for your future learning needs.

Considering your participation in the group today, list three ways you can improve your effectiveness in communicating your ideas, getting others to listen, explaining your viewpoint, or leading your group.

Ask a question on the current topic—a variation that causes the student to ponder another aspect.

From Glendon, K., & Ulrich, D. (1997). Unfolding cases: An experiential learning model. *Nurse Educator, 22,* 15–18. Reprinted with permission.

ing process help students learn more effectively than traditional methods. Yet these methods are not without problems for both faculty and student. In this new paradigm, the roles of both student and teacher change significantly, and it is inevitable that this drastic change in functioning will result in some frustration for both parties.

WHAT DO STUDENTS THINK?

If we are truly to evaluate this new paradigm, we need to address both the benefits and limitations of the strategies.

In analyzing our student evaluations from over 200 college students taking our classes that employed interactive methods, it was found that group strategies do have a multitude of student-recognized benefits. Only a few students noted specific frustrations as well. This analysis of student evaluations has helped us recognize limitations in our methods and design new approaches to overcome them.

Evaluation data were collected over an 18-month period through written and verbal comments. Students were asked to respond to open-ended questions, such as: "How do you feel about being in a class that uses group-learning strategies?" or "How do these strategies compare with the more traditional methods like lecture and discussion that you have experienced in other classes?" Also, specific strategies were listed, and students were asked to comment on each. In addition, the authors had focus groups or discussions with students as to the pros and cons and the effectiveness of these methods. Students were told at the beginning of the course that these were new and innovative strategies and that their opinions and reactions were very important to determine the usefulness of the strategies for student learning. Also, they were assured their reactions and perceptions would in no way affect their grade in the course.

Students' perceptions regarding our teaching methods fell into four positive and three negative themes. A few students reported negative feelings, but in most of the cases, students felt that the positive out-weighed the negative. Positive themes identified were the following:

1. *Increased understanding.* Students thought that the use of these group strategies helped them better understand the

material. Many stated that they thought they had to become involved and could not just sit back and daydream. This increased their understanding of the material and helped them learn and retain the material. Active involvement was identified as a factor essential to greater understanding.

2. *Enhancement of social interaction.* Numerous students commented on the social aspects of group learning. They felt "connected" to their group members and learned how to communicate their thoughts and ideas more effectively to others. They also enjoyed meeting new people and finding new friends.

3. *Encouragement of self-reflection.* Students were able to recognize that they were being exposed to new and different ideas and values. Because of some of the activities and discussions, they were made to look at opposing viewpoints and really examine and question their own value systems. Although most did not change their own ideas, they did think they could better appreciate the positions of others with different opinions.

4. *Promotion of group interdependence and responsibility.* Students overwhelmingly commented on their feelings of responsibility to their group. They recognized the change from a competitive arena to one of cooperation. Individual competitiveness seemed to be replaced with group caring. Students began to care about how others did and wanted to help their group do well.

The three negative themes were the following:

1. *Time commitment.* Some students thought that they were required to spend too much time on preparation and class activities. They thought that this took time away from the teacher preparing them for the test and telling them what was important to remember.

2. *Resentment of peer learning.* A handful of students resented "teaching themselves" and learning from their classmates. They thought the teacher was not doing the job that

he or she was being paid for, and that they should not have to pay to teach themselves.

3. *Ineffective groups.* A couple of students complained about their groups. They thought that they were put in a group that did not want to work or that had a few members who did not do their part. They thought it was unfair to them to have to work with people who could not function or chose not to function in the group-processing activities.

WHAT DO FACULTY THINK?

Students are not the only ones who cite negative consequences of group-learning strategies. Again, the literature overwhelmingly sings praises to the benefits of this new paradigm, and many faculty echo these praises; however, many other faculty members are finding it frustrating actually to implement these activities in their own classrooms. As human beings, we are all resistant to change, and many faculty members have a difficult time giving up the ways they are accustomed to teaching and the way they themselves were taught. Many feel awkward and uncomfortable at first or may have difficulty giving up the expert role and being the center of attention. Bevis (1989) relates that female nurse educators often have a difficult time relinquishing power as they have finally found a "voice" in our historically male-dominated culture and "are reluctant to give up this hard-won position." Also, many faculty members do not feel supported in trying new things and fear that their evaluation ratings will drop or that they will be criticized by administration or their colleagues for doing things differently from the norm. In addition, they fear students may react negatively when changes in teaching are implemented. Once they buy into the idea and actually implement the strategies, a whole new host of frustrations and questions emerge. How are groups formed? How are grades determined? How do I help groups interact socially as well as process tasks effectively? How can I assure that learning is actually occurring? They begin to face new problems that they are not used to and have no experience in solving. Often they revert back to their own comfort zone despite their beliefs that the new paradigm does result in a higher level of learning.

Faculty need to realize that there will be frustrations and problems as they begin working with groups. The best solution to these problems is to prevent them before they occur or have a plan to deal with the common issues inherent in interactive group learning. The following are common questions asked by faculty as they begin to implement interactive group learning.

How Can I Incorporate These New Group-Learning Strategies into My Present Lesson Plans?

Thinking about totally revamping and redoing lesson plans is overwhelming and is by no means necessary for the effective use of group-learning strategies. It is best to start slowly and become comfortable with the techniques before even thinking of using these methods extensively. Introduce the strategies one by one and begin implementing them in a class in which you feel very comfortable and have taught before. Use your old lesson plans, and add one new strategy at first. You might want to try a new strategy every week or every month to learn how to use them and then evaluate which strategies work best for you. If you are comfortable with the content, you will be better able to focus on the strategy and feel "safe" in experimenting with a new way of teaching familiar content. Do not feel you need to keep the students in the dark or make them think you are experienced in using these group methods. Share with them your reasons for trying them, and ask their assistance in helping you evaluate their effectiveness. Make them partners in your attempts to increase the effectiveness of their learning. If they feel a part of the plan, they are more apt to "buy into" a new way of thinking and learning as well as decrease their resistance and frustration with changes in methodology.

Also, allow yourself to fail, but keep trying. Not every strategy works with every class. You may experience several less than successful attempts before you really feel great about the effectiveness of a strategy. Find a colleague or group of colleagues and support each other as you all try to be more innovative and creative in your teaching. Share your successes and failures, and talk about ways to help students learn. Nothing stimulates faculty more than feeling free to brainstorm and talk about teaching. Change is difficult for all of us, yet we all want the best for our students. We need to support each other as we all grow as educators. Supporting one another builds collegiality and makes all of us better teachers.

Can These Strategies Be Used in Large Lecture Classrooms?

It certainly is easier to manage smaller classes physically when group-learning techniques are used, but it is entirely possible to use them in larger classes. As the instructor, you must make the class seem smaller and more intimate. This can be done by walking around the class as you talk, calling students by name, and interspersing cooperative group strategies that do not require a lot of movement or disruption. For example, you might say, "Find a partner, and using Think-Pair-Share, explain in your own words the concept I just discussed." In Think-Pair-Share, students have 1 minute think time after the teacher poses the question. Then, each student shares their answer with their partner. Selected pairs are asked to share their responses with the entire class. After having a few pairs report their explanation, you can assess how well the concept is understood and determine if it needs more attention to assure student learning. Students are active and involved despite the large class size. They feel connected to the content and each other.

Another idea is to use short writing assignments dealing with application of and reflection on course concepts, followed by a focused group discussion to help students feel involved with the content as well as involved with their peers. In general, any strategy can be used in a large class so long as the teacher thinks it through and modifies the strategy to fit the physical boundaries of the classroom and the time elements that must be adhered to. It is the teaching strategy, not the class size, that seems to determine learning outcomes (Bonwell & Eison, 1991). Try a variety of methods, including both in and out of class activities, that require students to collaborate with one another and become active in the process of learning. Large classes do not have to dictate a "lecture-only" method of teaching.

How Can I Grade Group Work on an Individual Basis?

Grading is a concern for both students and faculty and remains a continual problem for those of us who rely heavily on group activities in our classes. Using group grades alone is controversial and many faculty are rejecting it as an option. Students feel a loss of control in relation to the grade they receive if the entire group receives the same grade for various amounts of work contributed. They resent people who do nothing and still get the same grade as those who really put in time on the project. Other more reserved and quiet students resent those who dominate, take over, and do things without consulting others. One way to factor in these unacceptable behaviors is to use peer evaluation as the basis for individual evaluation. Every student grades each of the group members on a variety of things including the quality and quantity of their work, their social skills and group processing, and other elements inherent in group work (see Table 2.3 for an example). To prepare students for this evaluation, the professor must stress the importance of evaluating one's peers. Supportive comments, as well as the need for improvement, must be included. Participants must also have time to discuss the evaluation form, ask questions, and feel well informed on the things they are expected to do as group members. In this way, the peer evaluation will be fair and serve as a learning tool rather than a punitive activity. The faculty member averages the grades given to each individual student and that becomes part of that student's grade. In this way, students realize that if they do not function as effective group members, their grade will be affected. Students believe that group grades are fairer when this peer evaluation is used. Also, faculty can see who is carrying the brunt of the work load in the group and who is slacking.

TABLE 2.3   Peer Evaluation

Evaluate each member in your group, excluding yourself. In any case, when you give a 1 or 5, you must explain your reasoning in the comment section.

1 = Never; 2 = Rarely; 3 = Sometimes; 4 = Usually; 5 = Always

	Group Members:				
	1	2	3	4	5
1. I was satisfied with the quality of their work.					
2. I was satisfied with the quantity of their work.					
3. They attended all group meetings.					
4. They did their share of the work and contributed equally.					
5. They showed respect for all group members and used good group-processing skills.					

Totals:

Comments:

Faculty can also use a combination of group and individual grading in group activities. For example, if a group paper is submitted, students can be responsible for different parts of the paper. The faculty can grade each part individually and then the paper as a whole; each student would get an average of the two scores earned. Group presentations can be graded similarly, as a whole and individually for the part each student presents. In this way, collaboration and cooperation are essential, but people who do not do their part or do it in an inferior way are penalized in the grading process. Faculty who are concerned about the influence of groups' projects and papers inflating the individual student's grade require students to meet a minimum standard in all areas evaluated including individual objective testing. In this way, a student who falls below minimum standards on individual work could not pass a course because of the grade inflation from group grading.

What Do I Do About Absenteeism When Students Are Learning in Groups?

Absenteeism is a major problem and can hamper the effectiveness of group learning. To decrease it, faculty need to make students want to come to class. This can be accomplished in a variety of ways, such as taking off points from the final grade for missing classes, giving pop quizzes that cannot be made up, or collecting homework and grading it based on a coin toss each class period. Students almost always respond and attend class if not doing so affects their grade negatively. Also, once the group bonds and members realize that they hurt their group if they are absent, they feel responsible to be there. Peer pressure can also be called into play when students miss class consistently. In classes where group learning is the norm, professors can require attendance and drop people from the class if they miss more than three classes, for example. They can also figure attendance into the course grade. These practices, too, will keep absenteeism to a minimum.

What Do I Do if the Students in the Group Do Not Work Well Together?

This whole idea of groups not working well together is a major problem for students and faculty alike. Although it is not an overwhelming problem in most groups, you can count on having at least one group per class that develops some problems getting along and completing the task at hand. This can be extremely disruptive to the faculty member and the students in the group. The best way to handle this problem is to try to keep it from happening in the first place. Building in the following concepts will help prevent these problems from occurring.

The *initial forming of groups* is an important task for the professor and should be done in a very deliberate and organized manner.

In general, groups should consist of four to six members. In groups with fewer than four members, there are not enough ideas or opinions really to encourage critical thinking and problem solving. Groups of more than six are too difficult to control and work with. Too many ideas and opinions make coming to consensus or solving problems almost impossible. Heterogeneous groups are generally better in that there are more differences for students to experience. Groups should be heterogeneous for age, gender, race, ethnicity, academic abilities, special talents, and so on. In fact, it is often beneficial to administer survey questionnaires to determine learning style (Kolb, 1976) or personality characteristics (Myers & McCaulley, 1985) to assure even greater heterogeneity. The greater number of varying perspectives in a group makes more complete and effective team processing.

Team-building activities are also an important activity to prevent group problems. Although it may seem like a waste of class time to do this, it will prove to be a vital ingredient for an effective team. Teams that are enthusiastic and trust and respect each other will work better together and achieve greater academic success (Kagan, 1992; Solomon, Davidson, & Solomon, 1993). Group members need adequate time to get acquainted, develop identity as a team, learn to respect and value their differences, and feel a team bond. There are numerous things that can be done to help teams develop and feel a commitment to one another. One such activity that encourages members getting to know one another is "Guess the Fib" (Kagan, 1992). In this activity, each group member comes up with two true unbelievable facts about him- or herself and one believable fact that is not true. In turn, students state the three facts about themselves, and teammates guess which one is false. This activity helps students become better acquainted. To create a sense of team identity, teams might come up with a team name or logo. There are also many team-building exercises available for building respect for one another and for appreciating group differences, another needed element to assure group-processing effectiveness. "Bafa Bafa" (Hummel & Peters, 1994) is a game that can be played to help students see and respect different cultural values. Students are assigned to two fictional cultures. After learning the norms and values of their culture, they interact with the other group and try to figure out the norms of each other's culture. It is most effective in teaching differences for student nurses. Another activity, "Survival in the Desert," is an example of another structure that can be used to encourage respect for differences (Kagan, 1992). This activity challenges students to decide which items they would want to have if they were stranded in the desert. It requires group consensus and is an excellent team builder. Many more activities are available in recent literature. Taking the time for team building is essential for effective group functioning.

Teachers can also help students find reasons to value and respect others and even increase the self-esteem and participation of lower functioning or nonparticipating students by assigning competence to these low-status members. Cohen (1994) thinks that there is often a difference in the quality and level of participation of group members and that the more reserved and quiet students communicate a message of nonparticipation by their nonverbal and verbal actions, which further segregate them from those actively participating. Teachers can solve this dilemma in two distinct ways: first, by stressing that the group needs a variety of abilities to complete the task and that although no one student can possibly have all the necessary skills, everyone will have some of the skills necessary for success. Then, the teacher verbally acknowledges the specific skill the low-status student possesses. Perhaps the student is an expert computer programmer or a talented artist. The low-status student feels more competent, and others see what the student can offer to the group task (Cohen, 1994). In this way, the group will function more effectively as all group members will be involved and feel valued and respected.

Group rules and roles need to be established immediately after group formation. These can be assigned by the professor, determined by a group decision, or be a combination developed by both teacher and group. Rules might include a variety of things that must be adhered to by all group members. Rules might include the procedure that must be followed if a group decides to eliminate someone from the group for not contributing or being disruptive, and the consequences of not following the rules. Rules should be stated positively, be realistic, be easily understood, and be few in number. (See Table 2.4 for an example of common rules.) The

TABLE 2.4   Class Rules for Group Learning

1. All team members must participate and contribute their ideas and thoughts to the group.
2. Team members must work together and help each other. "One for all and all for one."
3. Team members must be prepared for every class by completing class assignments.
4. Team members must keep an open mind and listen to others' ideas and opinions.
5. Team members may criticize ideas but not people.
6. Team members may ask a group member to leave their group if they unanimously agree that that person is not abiding by the rules, they have informed the person that he or she is not meeting group expectations, and the entire team has had a conference with the instructor before the action.
7. Any member who has been asked to leave a group must either find another group to join; do the project individually, getting zero points for the peer evaluation and a maximum grade of C in the course; or drop the course.

use of assigned roles may also be used. The roles are usually rotated so each member gets an opportunity to function in all roles. Typical roles would include leader or task master, recorder, encourager, and substitute (see Table 2.5). Having rules and roles are essential structures that help teams function effectively.

Social skills development, including group skills and communication, is an important component of effective group functioning. Often students do not know how to work in groups. They have been

TABLE 2.5   Typical Group Roles

Team leader	Supervises team, gets group working, and assures that all participate; resolves conflicts (with help of other team members)
Recorder	Takes minutes; keeps records of all material, assignments, finished work, etc.; records members' absences; informs absent students of group activities
Task master	Keeps the team working toward the task at hand; intervenes if group gets off task and redirects their efforts
Substitute	Takes the role of any member absent

socialized to be competitive, not cooperative in their associations with peers. Before we can expect them to work as a team, we must teach them the skills they will need to carry out a cooperative group activity.

David and Roger Johnson have stressed the importance of groups defining and analyzing the roles members play (Kagan, 1992). They have identified "task roles" or the functions required in carrying out a group task. For a group to complete a task, it is essential that someone initiates the group activity and that group members give opinions, clarify information, elaborate on examples, and pull together their ideas. They also list "group-building and maintenance roles" or the functions required in strengthening and maintaining group life and activities. Behaviors of encouraging, mediating, relieving tension, and expressing group feelings are necessary functions that strengthen group cohesiveness. Other group maintenance roles that keep the group focused on the task are diagnosing, evaluating, choosing standards, and asking for group consensus. Additionally, they have identified nine types of non-functional behavior that do not help and can often hinder the group and the work the group is trying to accomplish. Some of these behaviors are blocking, withdrawing, being aggressive, and seeking sympathy. If groups are given this information and are aware of some of the principles of group dynamics, they can better identify and analyze the dynamics of their own group—hence, begin to have the knowledge to solve those problems or stop ineffective behaviors before they cause a group problem. Using mandatory individual and group evaluations helps students see how both they and their group members are functioning and can be used as the basis for group discussion of the group's effectiveness (see Table 2.6 for an example of such an evaluation form).

Other ways to help students learn how to function in a group could include the use of a "Group Grumbles Box." At the beginning of the first class, the teacher describes the use of the "Group Grumbles Box." It is a small covered closed box that sits outside the teacher's office. Any student can submit a group problem to the box for help in solving it. No names or information is to be used that will identify the group or the person causing the problem. Each week the faculty checks the box, and for the first few minutes

TABLE 2.6   Evaluation of Group Processing

	Never	Sometimes	Usually	Always

Self-Evaluation
I contributed my ideas freely.
I listened objectively to others' ideas.
I encouraged others to participate.
I was respectful of others.
I paid attention and stayed focused on
the task.
I avoided blaming, arguing, expressing
personal feelings, clowning, day-
dreaming, and other nonfunctional
behaviors.
When conflict occurred in the group, I
tried to mediate.
When conflict occurred, I helped the
group analyze the source of the diffi-
culty and what steps to take next.
When decisions were near, I asked for
group consensus.
Comments:

Evaluation of My Group
We worked well together and avoided
blaming, arguing, expressing personal feelings, clowning, day-
dreaming, and other nonfunctional
behaviors.
We stayed on task.
We respected and listened to each
other.
We encouraged and supported each
other.
When conflict occurred, we effectively
analyzed the difficulty and proceeded
with a plan to solve the conflict.
Group consensus occurred.
Decisions were evaluated and mea-
sured against our group goals.
Comments:

of class that day, a total class discussion evolves regarding how one should go about solving the problem at hand. If no problems are submitted, the teacher discusses a common problem, such as a group member who always has an excuse why he or she did not do the assigned part of the group project or a person who always insists things be done his or her way. These discussions give students experience in solving problems and give them concrete solutions to use if such problems occur in their group. It also makes everyone wonder which group or person submitted this problem and to whom it is referring, so if an individual thinks he or she may be the person being discussed, behavior may change before it causes a group problem. Students never know if the problem being discussed is one submitted by a peer or if it is teacher generated.

There are also several activities that groups can engage in to help them practice consensus building (see Table 2.7). One such activity is "You Have to Have a Heart" (Kagan, 1992). In this activity individuals first, and then in teams, prioritize from 1 to 5 which of five fictional characters should qualify for an artificial heart to save his or her life. As the teams try to come to consensus, they learn how to communicate their values and opinions and respect the differences of others. Yet, in the end, they must negotiate and come to consensus as a group.

TABLE 2.7   Rules for Making Decisions by Group Consensus

1. Group members will listen, with an open mind and without interrupting, while all members express their thoughts, ideas, and opinions.
2. Group members will not argue but will discuss differences of opinion.
3. Group members will remain open to modifying their own opinions as needed.
4. Group members will seek to gain at least some agreement of all group members.
5. Group members will not vote, bargain, or trade to reach a decision.
6. Group members will understand that reaching consensus will be time consuming but will result in all members feeling ownership of the final decision, which will increase its chance of success.

Other activities promote effective communication skills and allow students to practice these skills. In the activity "Island Maps" (Johnson, 1996) a deck of 30 cards is dealt face down among the group members. Each card in the set has an island shape drawn on it. There are matches for all but one island shape, and some islands have more than one match. The group must determine which card in the set is a single island. The rules state that the players can look only at the cards dealt to them, that they may not trade cards, they may not draw pictures or diagrams of the maps, they must keep their own discard piles, and they communicate according to established group rules. This activity requires the group to talk about the island shapes to complete the task of finding the single island card. The group that correctly identifies the single island card wins the game. It is a wonderful way for students to practice being specific and concise in their communication. These are skills necessary for effective group functioning.

If group problems occur despite efforts to avoid them, it is the teacher's responsibility first to diagnose the problem and then try to help students solve it. Often students need help in figuring out what the actual problem is, as they tend to focus on the symptoms of the problem rather than the cause. If it is the teacher who determines that a problem exists, it is her or his responsibility to alert the group to the concerns and together try to diagnose the cause of the problem in order to solve it. If student groups are required to keep group minutes, they can serve as a valuable tool to help diagnose problems and their cause. Minutes should include members present, times and places of meetings, group role assignments if they are being used, and assignments and due dates agreed on by the members. By reviewing minutes, faculty can help students pinpoint problem causes in some cases. The use of a peer evaluation as an intermittent check for all team members as well as a final evaluation tool can be useful in helping group members realize how their behaviors are being perceived by others. Often this alone will result in individuals changing their behaviors and solving the problem themselves. The bottom line in solving group problems is honest and open communication. Because students may not feel comfortable doing this or may not have the skill to do so, the teacher may have to facilitate and role model the appropriate ways to handle group conflict and problems.

How Do I Know How Much Time to Give Students to Process the Problems in the Group-Learning Activities?

Determining time limits for group activities is one of the most difficult things to do as there is no hard-and-fast rule. It is important to give students enough time to process adequately, yet not so much that they have extra time to socialize and "goof off." Experience is probably the best way to get a handle on this problem. When you first begin using group strategies, monitor time with a watch. Walk around the room and see how groups are coming along, ask one person in the group to stand when the group has finished processing the task, or ask one person to go to the board and write the group's solution when the group is finished. Soon you will have a better idea how much time to allot. The use of "Numbered Heads" (Kagan, 1992) promotes listening and active involvement in the group processing and is very effective as a tool in implementing group work and keeping everyone actively involved in the task (see Figure 2.2). Every student in the group is assigned a number before the activity. After the activity has been processed by the group, the teacher calls a number, and the person with that number in each group stands and gives the group's solution or goes to the board and writes the solution. Because students never know which number will be called, they are more likely to listen and stay involved. If everyone remains involved, time is used wisely.

What if I Am Ostracized for Trying New Ways by Both Fellow Faculty and Administration? Is It Worth It?

Nothing is more deflating to one's ego than being excited about a new way to teach and being "put down" for rocking the steady boat of tradition. To succeed, you need support, and if it is not there, you must actively create it! Find a buddy and help each

FIGURE 2.2   Numbered heads.

other as you both try to become better teachers. Meet frequently
to share your successes and failures, help each other devise ways
to use group-learning activities in your classes, develop a creative
strategy and publish it—nothing gets you more respect than being
published in a refereed journal! If the journal publishes it then
you have validation that it was a good idea, and you may find
former skeptical colleagues asking more about your new methods.
Perhaps volunteering to be on the faculty development committee
will put you in a position to educate your faculty on this new
education paradigm. You can encourage them to attend education
conferences and read education journals, or you might circulate
a new educational strategy from your favorite journal each month.
If possible, encourage your department to hire a consultant to
help everyone see the value in these group methods and help them
integrate these strategies into your specific curriculum. Change is
inevitable, and in time, we will all be expected to teach in accor-
dance with this new paradigm, so let's embrace the change and
not resist it!

How Do I Deal with Students Who Complain That They Are Teaching Themselves?

This is a common comment from students who are used to and accept traditional ways of learning. As with faculty, you must educate them as to the benefits of this new paradigm and win them over to at least giving the new way a chance. Tell them about what you are doing and why, and ask for their suggestions and evaluation of the strategies. Explain the new paradigm (see Table 1.1), and ask them to experiment with the new ways. Try to explain that you are trying to teach them how to think and problem solve, and reassure them that they will learn and retain more if they apply information as is required in group-processing tasks. We need to help our students move from dualistic to multiplistic thinking (Perry, 1970). Thinking is a developmental process in which students make the transition from viewing the world in black and white to understanding that the world is really shades of gray.

What Do I Do if Student Groups Generate Unsatisfactory or Incomplete Solutions?

The key to student group processing is preparation before class. If students do not have basic information about the concepts and content relevant to the group task, they cannot possibly be successful in completing it. Homework in the form of study guides (see Table 2.1) or open-ended reflective-writing prompts (see Table 2.2) are necessary for students to complete before class and must reflect important and relevant information to be used in classroom activities. In this way, they have had the opportunity to read about and try to understand whatever the topic of the class is before class time and are better prepared to ask questions and apply facts to typical nursing situations and problems. Class time, while the teacher is present, is the time students should work on application of facts and information, as the teacher can serve as a resource person and facilitator. Using class time to repeat reams of facts that are in a book is a waste of the short time students have to interact with the teacher and their peers. Again, teaching is not telling. Once students realize that they cannot actively participate in the group activities if they are not prepared, they tend to come to class ready to work, and your problems are solved. One way to assure this preparation is to check study guides periodically or give students points for doing them. A crossword puzzle, used individually or as a group, could be a quick check to assure that students are familiar with pertinent terms relevant to the class topic (see Chapter 5). These methods help students become more self-disciplined in preparing and processing tasks in class. Also, an important teacher responsibility is to clarify information, correct misconceptions, and summarize the important points after the group activity. In this way, the teacher can assess students' understanding and competence in this particular area. If it is apparent that students are not grasping the necessary knowledge, the teacher can try a new teaching strategy to illustrate the missing knowledge. All of these tips can help assure effective student task resolution.

I Don't Like the Feeling of "No Control" I Feel When I Use These Methods, and I Don't Feel I Am Covering All of the Material

First of all, realize that your feelings are normal ones. We all teach like we were taught, and we all resist change, especially if we feel we are doing a good job teaching in a traditional way. Before you will feel comfortable with the new methods, you must give them a chance. You need to accept the new paradigm and admit to yourself that teaching is not telling and that memorization of facts is not real learning. Try to integrate one group strategy into your lesson plan once a week and then increase it as you become more comfortable. In time, you will adjust to being more spontaneous and realize that the classroom is not out of control at all; rather, it is structured chaos, and you are the one who structured it! You will soon feel more secure in not being able to answer every question they may have and feel good about showing them how to find the answers to their own questions in books, on the Internet, and by calling resource people. You are giving them the skills to solve their own problems, not only an answer to a question.

Covering content is another real worry for teachers. We feel obligated to tell students everything we know, and we still feel that the only way to teach is to tell. Again, we must change our assumptions about what teaching is and what learning is. We cover content in a new way, by asking students to read and prepare at home using study guides and then to apply the information in class group activities. One way to assure yourself that you are, in fact, covering the content is to use a variety of classroom assessment techniques (Angelo & Cross, 1993; Cross & Angelo, 1988; Cross & Steadman, 1996). Techniques like the "1-minute paper" can help you validate that you are, in fact, teaching students the content they need, just in a different and more effective way. In this technique, students are asked to take one minute to answer a question posed by the faculty member. By asking them to explain a difficult concept or apply one to a clinical situation you, the instructor, can determine the learning that has occurred.

Yet another issue plagues all of us as nurse educators. What content should we teach? This question is more complex than is readily apparent. What knowledge is essential for students before asking them to think and process critically? As a profession, we have several levels of nurses, LPN, ADN, BSN, MSN, and PhD. The knowledge that each requires differs in both breadth and depth. It is this very issue that perplexes faculty. First as a profession and then as teachers for these various groups of students, we need to determine appropriate learning outcomes for each of the levels. Once this is done, the subsequent problem of overwhelming students with impossible reams of information without helping them discriminate essential knowledge will be eased. However, it may be some time before the nursing profession details those delineations; with the knowledge and technology explosion facing society today, it is apt to remain a continued concern for all of us. In the meantime, you must decide for yourself what is most important and design study guides using focused questions that will help the student concentrate on the important facts.

SUMMARY

These are many of the questions faculty ask as they begin to implement these new ideas. It is hoped that the comprehensive group learning model and discussion of frequently asked questions will ease your transition to group learning and ultimately enhance the learning potential of your students as well as stimulate you to continue to broaden your repertoire of teaching techniques. Using these interactive methods will broaden students' abilities to communicate and work together with peers of different cultures, ages, genders, and mental/physical abilities. These are skills they will use in the work world where understanding the complexity of diversity is paramount.

CHAPTER 3

Using Cooperative-Learning Strategies in Nursing

Cooperative-learning strategies are specific group-learning structures that help the faculty require students to be active participants in the learning process. These structures can be used individually or combined, as the only method of teaching, or as a break from traditional lecture methods. This chapter discusses several cooperative strategies for teachers to experiment with.

THINK-PAIR-SHARE

Think-Pair-Share is a simple classic cooperative-learning strategy developed by Frank Lyman (1987). It involves all students and is quick and easy to implement in any class, be it a seminar of 12 or lecture hall of 100. The professor poses a problem or question. Each student is given 60 seconds of "think" time, then students share their ideas or thoughts about the answers to the question or problem with a peer (see Figure 3.1). At that point, each pair may report the solution to the entire class, or selected pairs may be called on randomly to share solutions.

Using this strategy allows students time to process the task individually before sharing it with another student. Everyone must be involved, and no one is permitted to sit passively. On sharing

Think   **Pair and Share**

FIGURE 3.1   Cooperative strategy: Think, pair, and share.

their individual solutions with another student, students get both positive reinforcement and support for their answer, which increases their confidence before presenting their thoughts to the whole class. Students get practice in presenting their solutions to the class, which enhances the development of their communication skills. This not only decreases their anxiety but builds their self-esteem. An additional benefit is the increased depth of learning that occurs when students must explain their ideas or solutions to another student. This requires them to analyze their own thinking processes thoroughly, an important aspect of critical thinking and reflecting. During the whole class discussion following pairs reporting to the class, professors have the chance to correct misconceptions and assess students' depth of comprehension.

A professor might use this strategy to determine if students truly understand a complex situation or concept. For example, the professor could be lecturing on a topic such as Rh incompatibility. After the professor completes the explanation, he or she might ask students to first think about how they might explain this concept to a student who missed the class. After one minute of "think time," the students, in turn, explain the concept to their partners. After sharing their ideas, the professor calls on random pairs to stand and share their explanations. This gives the professor the opportunity to correct misconceptions immediately, assess the clarity of students' understanding, and reinforce the major points.

This strategy can also be used as an assessment tool periodically to ascertain student questions related to the content being presented or as a quick way to make a traditional lecture more interactive. Total time for this strategy can be as little as five minutes, depending on how many student pairs are called on to report. It could also be modified to include writing to give students practice in communicating. In this case, students would "think," then put their thoughts on paper or "write," and then "pair" and "share." Students could read and react to each other's written thoughts, helping each understand the strengths and limitations in the ability to communicate through writing.

ROUNDTABLE

Roundtable (Kagan, 1992) is a classic cooperative-learning strategy used primarily for brainstorming. Students are assigned to a group and sit in a circular fashion while a pad of paper is passed from one student to the next. Each student verbalizes and records a possible response to the problem or question proposed by the teacher, then passes the paper to the next student. One person is then called on to report for the entire group (see Figure 3.2). It

FIGURE 3.2   Cooperative strategy: Roundtable.

is very important that students both respond in turn and verbalize their thoughts. This prevents one or two members of the group from dominating the other members of the group and requires that everyone must participate. No one can just sit and listen. By responding verbally, each group member hears the others' ideas and can become stimulated by those ideas, the ultimate purpose of this brainstorming exercise. One benefit of this strategy is that students soon realize the importance of preparation before coming to class as they know that they will be required to participate. Faculty members need to be sure to inform students of the content to be covered either verbally or through the syllabus, so that preparation is possible. Another benefit of working in this roundtable structure is that it encourages students to communicate with one another and helps them to begin to work in teams. Students learn important communication and social skills, such as how to include others who are often quiet in discussion, the value of hearing everyone's ideas, and the need to respect others.

Roundtable is simple to use yet produces large volumes of information. In nursing classes, instead of lecturing on signs and symptoms of a particular disease, such as increased intracranial pressure, the professor could ask students to brainstorm a list of possible signs and symptoms. Students can individually think of a couple of signs, but a long list of signs is usually formulated when students are asked to do this as a group. Once student groups report to the whole class, most signs and symptoms are reported, but if they are not, faculty can add any signs or correct signs that were not appropriate. During this roundtable technique, students often feel free to ask more questions because they are stimulated by the discussion, and the technique itself invites and creates an open environment.

PASS THE PROBLEM

Pass the Problem (Kagan, 1992) usually begins with the roundtable technique in which students, in a group, process a problem or task by writing their ideas down on a sheet of paper in turn. Once their ideas are jotted down, the paper is then passed to another group of students (see Figure 3.3). When each group has a new set of ideas or solutions, the members are required to clarify, prioritize, add more solutions, or whatever the teacher proposes. At this point, student groups report their solutions or they can Pass the Problem again. With the previous example, students were required to list the signs and symptoms of increased intracranial pressure. Once each group listed all of its ideas, the list is passed to another student group. The new student group could be asked to clarify the list to be sure that these are, in fact, signs of increased intracranial pressure. They could add additional signs to the list, or a teacher might ask them to identify the early and late signs of increased intracranial pressure from the list they have been passed. Reporting of these signs and symptoms, such as restlessness, vomiting, headache, pupillary changes, and Cushing's phenomena, adds to their ability to remember this factual information. When reporting their group's ideas, it also increases their understanding of priority signs and emphasizes the importance of knowing the significance of particular signs. In this example, a student might indicate that changes in level of consciousness indicate an early sign of intracranial pressure, whereas vital sign changes often indi-

FIGURE 3.3   Cooperative strategy: Pass the problem.

cate late signs or brainstem herniation. Through this technique students gain ideas from the previous group's brainstorming efforts and must analyze and use their powers of critical thinking to process the task.

FORMULATE-SHARE-LISTEN-CREATE

Formulate-Share-Listen-Create is a cooperative structure formulated by Johnson, Johnson, and Smith (1991). In this structure a group of students is assigned a question or problem. First, students individually formulate an answer to the question/problem posed by the faculty member. In turn each student verbalizes his or her answer as other group members actively listen. Then the group as a whole creates a new answer incorporating the best ideas from each of the individual members. For example, in a class on growth and development the faculty might pose the problem a mother has with her unruly 2-year-old. The mother fears he will be hurt as he does not listen, runs wildly about, throws things, and climbs fearlessly on furniture in public and at home. Students would be asked to devise a solution that could be shared with the mother. Each student individually comes up with an idea that is shared with the group. Using the combined solutions developed the group formulates a new creative approach to share with the mother. This structure promotes active listening and gives each member equal voice as the problem is solved. It is particularly valuable when groups are relying only on one or two members' ideas to complete the assignment.

JIGSAW

Jigsaw (Aronson, Blaney, Stephen, Sikes, & Snapp, 1978) is a versatile group-learning structure that presents information on a variety of related concepts. Jigsaw not only encourages students to study nursing content but also provides the opportunity for students to use the critical thinking skills of analysis, reflection, synthesis, and reconstruction (see Figure 1.3). These skills are best integrated through a cooperative-learning experience. The following example using a Jigsaw illustrates the use of these important skills (Ulrich & Glendon, 1995).

Individual students are assigned one specific nursing theory. For example, students number off from 1 to 4, and each number is assigned a different theorist. After researching and analyzing their assigned theory individually before class, students group and interact with other students who were assigned the same theory (see Figure 3.4, above the arrow). The main focus of this group's assignment is to become "experts," which requires them to answer several questions and explore a variety of concepts regarding the topic, in this case, a specific nursing theory. These questions are formulated by the professor and based on pertinent facts necessary

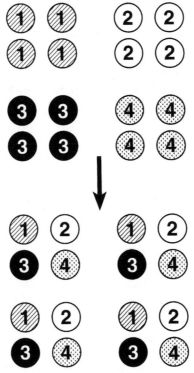

FIGURE 3.4   Cooperative strategy: Jigsaw.

to grasp the essence of the topic being studied. Group interaction is facilitated by using specific group learning structures. In this example, terminology used by the theorist, major concepts, application, and limitations are areas in which students must become knowledgeable to comprehend the theory.

Once students have become experts on their theory, they are regrouped so that there is one expert per theory in the new groups (see Figure 3.4, below the arrow). Each group member, in turn, explains his or her theory to the members of the new group so that all members become knowledgeable about each theory. Then the group creates a new theory based on knowledge gained from existing theories. The final step involves each group sharing its new theory with the entire class. See Table 3.1 for a summary of all the steps of Jigsaw.

This technique promotes several critical thinking concepts. Initially, students must prepare individually, learning facts, analyzing the theory, and explaining their ideas and interpretation of the theory to others. This sharing activity encourages other group members to reflect on their own ideas and to question others' perspectives. During this process, each student's understanding of the theory is enhanced through exposure to the ideas of others. When new groups form, students gain experience in teaching

TABLE 3.1   Steps in Jigsaw

Jigsaw 1	Students study individually their assigned nursing theory before class. Students who are assigned the same theory meet and discuss pertinent knowledge relative to the theory.
Jigsaw 2	New groups are formed consisting of at least one person from each theory group. Individual members explain their theory to the other members of the group so that all members become knowledgeable about each theory.
Jigsaw 3	Using the comprehensive knowledge gained through Jigsaw 2, the group creates a new theory.
Jigsaw 4	Each group presents its theory to the entire class. Discussion follows.

From Ulrich, D., & Glendon, K. (1995). Jigsaw: A critical thinking experience. *Nurse Educator*, *20*, 6–7. Reprinted with permission.

others. Students must synthesize the information gained through the previous group experience and articulate this information to the new group. Finally, as the new groups develop their own theory, synthesis of all theories culminates in a reconstruction of concepts into a newly developed theory. This final step relies on knowledge of other theories but also requires students to think imaginatively.

There are numerous ways Jigsaw could be used in the nursing classroom. For example, in a management class, various ways that nursing care is delivered could be explored using this method. Groups become experts on team nursing, primary care, and case management, and ultimately design a new creative approach to care giving. As students explore the advantages and disadvantages to quality care, the cost of each method, the patient outcomes, the required patient–nurse ratio, as well as the RN and health care worker mix required, they are able to analyze methods used in nursing practice critically.

Even nursing didactic content could be taught using Jigsaw. Individuals become experts on one type of diabetes (types 1 and 2, and gestational), and then teach it to new group members using the frame work of diet, exercise, and medication. Instead of Jigsaw 3, as shown in Table 3.1, students could find similarities and differences of the various kinds of diabetes, encouraging them to compare and contrast the various types. The variations are endless.

Jigsaw is a creative teaching strategy that promotes individual responsibility and group interdependence. It requires students to think critically and creatively, skills essential to practicing professional nursing. It truly meets the learning outcomes inherent in the new learning paradigm.

INSIDE-OUTSIDE CIRCLE

Inside-Outside Circle (Kagan, 1992) has many uses. It can be a structure used for team building and getting acquainted with team members or the entire class. It can be used as preparation for applying information in group class activities, reviewing for an examination, or as a means of memorizing and remembering important facts. In these situations, it is almost like a game in that students learn while moving about and having fun.

Students form two equal circles (i.e., 10 students in one circle and 10 in the other). The circles form so that one circle is inside the other one (see Figure 3.5). Students in the inside circle face outward and students in the outside circle, inward. As the circles form, each student is facing a partner. The teacher poses a factual question, such as "When do pregnant mothers experience quickening?" The pair discusses and comes to consensus on the answer. If they don't know the answer, they can ask the pair beside them. After 30 to 45 seconds the teacher rings a bell and asks for the answer. When everyone knows the correct answer, in this case, 20 weeks, the teacher says "rotate." Inside-circle members rotate clockwise, and outside-circle members rotate counterclockwise. Each student has a new partner, and the process repeats itself.

A variation would be to give each student a 3 × 5 card, with a question on one side and the answer on the other. When they pair, they ask their partner the question on the card, praise the

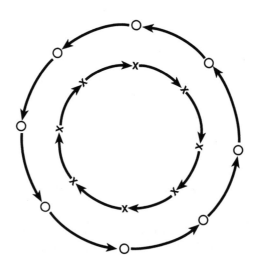

Inside circle rotates clockwise
Outside circle rotates counterclockwise

FIGURE 3.5   Inside-outside circle.

partner if he or she answers correctly, and show the answer if the partner is incorrect or does not know. Before rotating, students exchange cards. The process repeats until everyone has seen all the questions.

ACADEMIC CONTROVERSY

Academic Controversy (Johnson & Johnson, 1984) is an excellent group strategy that uses intellectual conflict as the basis for learning. It is similar to a traditional debate, except that students are forced to look at both sides of an issue, not just one side. It involves analysis of the issue as well as critical thinking to find a solution to rationalize agreement with one side or the other.

The teacher selects an important intellectual issue (see Table 3.2 for examples that might be used in nursing situations). Students are put into groups of four, with two being assigned the pro position and two the con position. Then, the five-step controversy procedure described by Johnson and Johnson (1984) is followed. First, the pairs are given time to research their topic and find the best reasons for supporting their assigned position. They also plan a way to present their position to persuade the opposing pair to their side. Second, each pair presents the case to the opposing pair. Third,

TABLE 3.2   Possible Nursing Topics for Academic Controversy

1. Assisted suicide is an accepted solution for consenting adults, and nurses should help if asked.
2. Fathers should have a legal right to a child before a mother chooses abortion, and if he wants the child, the mother's abortion should be denied.
3. Marijuana should be a legalized medicine as a schedule 1 drug.
4. Chemically dependent nurses should be able to practice.
5. Homosexual couples should be able to adopt children.
6. In vitro fertilization and other expensive fertility treatments should be paid for by insurance companies.
7. Organ donation should be an automatic procedure for everyone unless people have a legal document stating their objection.
8. Human cloning should be legalized.

in an open debate, the issue is discussed, critically evaluated, and defended by each side. Fourth, the two pairs reverse sides and present the best argument for the opposing position. Fifth, the four students drop their identified sides and discuss the issue objectively. They integrate the "best" of both sides and decide with which side they agree.

The benefits of this activity are many. Students are able to examine an issue from different perspectives and are forced to examine critically their own values and ideas for rationality. Research has consistently shown that this group activity promotes higher achievement, higher academic self-esteem, and higher quality problem-solving skills (Johnson & Johnson, 1984, 1989; Johnson, Johnson, & Smith, 1998; Millis & Cottell, 1998).

TEACHING NURSING CONTENT BY COMBINING STRATEGIES

As described by Glendon and Ulrich (1992a), the teaching plan shown in Tables 3.3 to 3.6 describes how nursing content can be taught cooperatively using multiple cooperative-learning strategies. Table 3.3 identifies the content to be covered, time allotment, and the specific student and teacher preparation before class. The student completes the assigned readings or audiovisual aid related to the topic. The teacher divides the class into heterogeneous groups of four to six members and decides on the specific cooperative strategy to be used. The teacher also determines the reward for group participation and designates the grading system.

Table 3.4 describes the first cooperative strategy, Think-Pair-Share, used to identify the defining characteristics of a particular condition, pregnancy-induced hypertension (PIH). This strategy allows students time to process the task and share their thoughts with another student. When the student receives positive reinforcement from a peer that high blood pressure, protein in the urine, and weight gain are the cardinal defining characteristics of PIH, confidence in participating in subsequent class discussion is enhanced. Table 3.5 explains a second cooperative strategy, Roundtable, which is used to brainstorm possible nursing diagnoses.

TABLE 3.3   Preparation

Content: Pregnancy-Induced Hypertension (PIH)

Student Preparation

1. Read Chapter 29, "Hypertensive States of Pregnancy," in your maternity textbook.
2. Complete the interactive videodisc on "Pregnancy-Induced Hypertension" in the computer center.

Teacher Preparation

1. Planning of assignments as stated previously.
2. Divide class into heterogeneous groups of four members and determine cooperative-learning strategies to be used.

    - Think-Pair-Share produces the defining characteristics (15 minutes).
    - Roundtable generates nursing diagnoses (15 minutes).
    - Pass the Problem brainstorms possible nursing interventions (20 minutes).

3. Teacher will quiz one member of each group and award two bonus points to each group member's next individual test grade, if answered correctly.

From Glendon, K., & Ulrich, D. (1992a). Using cooperative learning strategies. *Nurse Educator, 17*, 37–40. Reprinted with permission.

TABLE 3.4   Steps in Think-Pair-Share

- Ask students to list the defining characteristics of PIH while in their learning groups.
- Teacher allows 1 minute for each student to think individually about the defining characteristics.
- Two minutes are allowed for students to share thoughts with each other.
- Five minutes are allowed for both pairs to share thoughts with each other.
- A group list of defining characteristics evolves.
- Each group reports.
- Teacher creates a class list of defining characteristics, adding any missed items if necessary; stimulates discussion of pathophysiology and variation of disease process.

From Glendon, K., & Ulrich, D. (1992a). Using cooperative learning strategies. *Nurse Educator, 17*, 37–40. Reprinted with permission.

TABLE 3.5   Steps in Roundtable

- Using the class list of defining characteristics, each group is asked to generate a list of possible nursing diagnoses.
- Brainstorming is facilitated by requiring each student to generate a diagnosis. A pad of paper is passed in turn to each student.
- After 10 minutes, one member of each group is asked to report the diagnoses on their group list to the class.
- The teacher lists the diagnoses on the board or an overhead transparency as each group reports, suggests missed diagnoses, and promotes general discussion.

Glendon, K., & Ulrich, D. (1992a). Using cooperative learning strategies. *Nurse Educator*, *17*, 37–40. Reprinted with permission.

Roundtable encourages each student to analyze a defining characteristic of PIH, such as elevated blood pressure. Then, students determine a valid nursing diagnosis for the characteristic—in this case, potential for injury related to a possible convulsion. The ability to link the defining characteristic to the appropriate nursing diagnosis is difficult for beginning nursing students, and this exercise provides the opportunity to practice this essential skill. Students soon realize the importance of preparation before class, as the strategy requires them to participate actively in turn. No one can just sit back and listen. However, the group that is practicing social skills tolerates error and creates an environment of acceptance, freeing students to participate actively.

Table 3.6 discusses yet a third specific cooperative technique, Pass the Problem, which generates nursing interventions specific to the nursing diagnoses previously defined. Pass the Problem allows the first group of students to brainstorm a list of interventions related to a specific nursing diagnosis, such as potential for injury related to a possible convulsion. This list generally includes the obvious interventions, such as monitoring blood pressure and reflexes, administering magnesium sulfate, and instituting seizure precautions.

When passed to the second group, they add to, refine, and clarify the list. They often include additional parameters related to the blood pressure, for example, to call the physician if the

TABLE 3.6   Steps in Pass the Problem

- Each group selects one nursing diagnosis.
- Teacher creates a folder for each selected nursing diagnosis and gives one folder to each group.
- Each group generates as many possible interventions in 10 minutes, writing interventions on paper provided in folder.
- The new group adds to and refines the existing list of interventions, creating a new list by writing on an overhead transparency provided in the folder.
- Each group reports the list of interventions related to a specific diagnosis.
- The teacher promotes discussion as the interventions are presented, suggesting interventions, and/or refining and clarifying the list.

From Glendon, K., & Ulrich, D. (1992a). Using cooperative learning strategies. *Nurse Educator, 17,* 37–40. Reprinted with permission.

blood pressure is greater than 160/100 and to position the patient on her left side. Additional interventions of measuring intake and output and assessing daily weight gains are usually identified by this second group because they must reflect on more specific details of the condition.

At the end of each strategy, the groups report their results, and the teacher verifies that the information is complete. The caliber of discussion proceeds at a higher level as students have been immersed in the material and have had time to think and reflect on the content presented.

This example, pregnancy-induced hypertension, explains how nurse educators might teach course content using multiple cooperative-learning strategies rather than traditional lecture. Essential content can be taught employing these methods, while at the same time encouraging critical thinking and practicing communication techniques in teams. Students have the opportunity to "discover" knowledge rather than "receive" it from faculty. They are active, involved, and feel connected to the material—all characteristics that promote more effective learning.

This chapter described specific cooperative-learning strategies that are used to stimulate group interaction and problem solving. Faculty members can use these strategies alone or in combination to meet their individual student-learning needs in both the classroom and clinical areas.

CHAPTER 4

Using the "Unfolding Case Model"

Educators today are realizing the value of designing strategies that actively involve students for outcomes of the new learning paradigm. Nurse educators in particular are aware of the need to prepare student nurses for managing clients with various needs in an environment driven by demands of cost containment and managed care plans. The reality is that data are often complicated and continually changing as clients' health status improves or declines and as information is obtained from other health care providers, clients, and their families. Rarely does the nurse know the whole picture before care. With shortened hospital stays, the nurse must obtain, analyze, and synthesize available data about the patient and plan nursing care accordingly. This requires an experienced level of critical thinking and communicating. Our "Unfolding Cases" (Glendon & Ulrich, 1997, 2001) design meets the goal of actively involving students as well as allowing them practice time to individually, as well as collectively, solve problems they may encounter in clinical situations. The net effect is a greater repertoire of skills and perspectives to apply when faced with new problems and challenges.

As described by Glendon and Ulrich (1997, 2001), "Unfolding Cases" is a variation and extension of the frequently used strategy of case studies (Dailey, 1992). It presents an ever-changing case or scenario that students process sequentially. An "Unfolding Case" usually contains three paragraphs, although individual educators could design as many additional paragraphs as they need to meet their learning goals. The first paragraph sets the stage for the scenario. It includes pertinent background information related to the characters of the case, the initial situation they find themselves in, and focused questions. Groups of students interact to process the focused questions and then share their interactions with the entire class. To facilitate discussion and interaction among peers, cooperative-learning strategies, such as *Roundtable* (Kagan, 1992), *Think-Pair-Share* (Lyman, 1987), and *Pass the Problem* (Kagan, 1992), are used (Glendon & Ulrich, 1992a). Then, the second paragraph is revealed. This paragraph could reflect a change in time, build on the last paragraph, or include a new focus. Students again process the questions of this paragraph and share the findings through cooperative-learning exercises. At this point, any further paragraphs are sequentially revealed, building on the case, or changing its focus. The final step is an individual reflective writing exercise that could encourage students to plan for their future learning needs, to think about and share individual reactions, or to reflect on and thus deepen the learning experience.

In building the structure of the case, the professor needs to address seven specific areas: purpose of the case, biographical data, context, content, focused questions, cooperative-learning strategies, and reflective writing. In the *purpose of the case* professors must first clarify the intent of this exercise, or what it is they want the students to gain from participating in the case. Is this case to be used for one entire class, a series of classes, or as a post-clinical wrap-up session? What are the expected outcomes? Is it to teach content or apply previously learned concepts? Professors need to plan expected answers to augment discussion when needed and to ensure all pertinent information is discussed.

The case example in Table 4.1 was designed with many purposes in mind. One of the purposes was to allow students the opportunity to apply assessment findings to the pathophysiology of heart defects. The given set of data indicated some of the classic signs of cardiac disease in children, which included low weight, history of respiratory illness, and clinical signs of dyspnea on exertion, fatigue, cyanosis, and clubbing of the fingers. The professor would expect students to investigate further clinical signs, such as

TABLE 4.1   Case Example for Nursing Education

Learning Outcomes

After processing the case, the student will be able to

- Apply assessment findings to pathophysiology of heart defects.
- Apply principles of preoperative and postoperative nursing care for a cardiac catheterization.
- Plan individualized discharge teaching for the client/family.
- Use resources for identified problems.

Paragraph 1

Day 1, 0800: Molly is a 10-year-old Caucasian girl admitted to Children's Hospital with cardiomyopathy. She has been seen several times in recent years for pneumonia. A cardiac catheterization is planned for tomorrow. Her weight is 27.7 kg. The night nurse indicates in report that Molly has dyspnea on exertion and tires easily. She also has circumoral cyanosis and clubbing of the fingers.

Focused Questions and Cooperative-Learning Strategies

Group 1	Relate the current clinical data to child's diagnosis. What data are important to collect considering the child's diagnosis and symptoms? What would you expect to find?	**Roundtable**
Group 2	What standardized teaching is included in preoperative and postoperative preparation for a cardiac catheterization? How would you individualize this teaching for a 10-year-old child?	**Roundtable**
Group 3	Develop and prioritize a list of nursing diagnoses for Molly followed by three nursing interventions for each diagnosis.	**Roundtable**
		After all three groups have finished, each group must pass the problem to another group. Each group processes a new list of nursing diagnoses and interventions, refining and adding more to the list; groups report their findings.

(continued)

TABLE 4.1   *(continued)*

Paragraph 2

Day 2, 0930, cardiac catheterization: The child returns from the procedure. Her color remains dusky around the lips. RR18, no retracting of nasal flaring noted. Bp WNL. R femoral site has dressing saturated with bright red blood. Peripheral pulses are strong and equal.

Focused Questions and Cooperative Learning Strategies

Pairs of students	What could be happening with the introduction of this new data? What data are needed to support your conclusion? What do you do if you decide there are abnormalities?	**Think-Pair-Share** Pairs are called on to report.

Paragraph 3

Discharge day: Instructions are written as follows: Home O_2 therapy at night. Protimes once per week. Medications of digoxin 0.125mg q12 hours po and captopril 12.5 mg po q8 hours. You already called the company that supplies home O_2 therapy and find the family has been denied service because of a lack of insurance. You find out mom is not on welfare. In your interactions with mom yesterday, she confides to you that she has a "nervous" problem and takes numerous medications that cost a lot of money. Mom also needs frequent reminding related to the child's needs, and you are beginning to wonder if she is capable of following a medication schedule for Molly.

Focused Questions and Cooperative Learning Strategies

Groups 1–3	Considering our role as coordinator of care, how would you plan for discharge? What course of action is indicated with the addition of new data related to mom? Consider the options and decide on the best approach.	**Roundtable. Report each group's findings.**

Reflective-Writing Prompt

Suppose that when you reported excessive bleeding to the physician after the cardiac catheterization, the physician responded with, "lots of kids bleed, don't worry about it." How would you feel, and what would you do?

From Glendon, K., & Ulrich, D. (1997). Unfolding cases: An experiential learning model. *Nurse Educator, 22,* 15–18. Reprinted with permission.

oxygen saturation, respiratory rate, need for oxygen, adventitious lung sounds, heart murmur, heart rate and rhythm, peripheral pulses, capillary refill, peripheral edema, and hematocrit. Students are challenged to apply knowledge of data given as well as data missing, and the professor must be prepared to clarify and add to the discussion.

Biographical data on all characters of the case need to be created. Information, such as age, sex, culture, socioeconomic status, and educational level, needs to be included. Such information brings the case to life, highlighting the individuality of the client situation. In this specific case, a 10-year-old white child, her mother, and a nurse are identified. Paragraph one of the case includes information one might find in a chart or kardex as well as some assessment data obtained from the night nurse (see Table 4.1).

Context refers to several different aspects, such as environment, historical information, resources available, or the situation at hand. Context could also refer to biographical information, such as a person's gender, cultural perspective, or frame of reference. The content of the case example occurs in the hospital, beginning with admission data and moving to planning for discharge. The example case highlights the situation the nurse is faced with when bleeding occurs post–cardiac catheterization (see Table 4.1).

Content includes a variety of concepts, such as pathophysiology, treatments, medications, health promotion and prevention concepts, legal and ethical issues, laboratory findings, teaching, and discharge planning as seen in the case example (see Table 4.1). These concepts represent the knowledge that students must be able to apply in clinical situations and are often the focus of the questions asked of the student groups.

Focused questions are used to encourage students to brainstorm and problem solve the issues inherent in the case. These questions are designed to stimulate critical thinking related to the nurse educator's learning outcomes. Typical questions might direct students to evaluate information given in the case, or may require them to anticipate expected findings from their previous knowledge (Browne & Keeley, 1990). In the case example, students were asked to apply knowledge of pathophysiology to plan appropriate nursing interventions for Molly. Questions may even ask students to identify pros and cons of an intervention or course of action. Students in the case explore what to do about bleeding post–cardiac catheterization (see Table 4.1).

Strategies used in processing the case are based on cooperative learning principles. A key benefit of cooperative learning is that it encourages students to communicate with their peers. The ability to articulate their ideas is enhanced in this interactive process. Students realize that having to explain a concept to someone else ensures understanding and enhances their own memory. Some strategies that work well include *Think-Pair-Share* (Lyman, 1987), *Roundtable* (Kagan, 1992), and *Pass the Problem* (Kagan, 1992), to name a few, although additional cooperative strategies could be used (Ulrich & Glendon, 1994, 1995). Because the professor assigns each student group a separate question to process, groups work individually on their tasks and ultimately share results with the entire class. As students stand and report their group's ideas, confidence is gained in communicating with others, yet another benefit of the exercise.

Reflective writing is used to complete the entire exercise. It serves as a method of encouraging individual student reflection on the learning that has occurred, gives students something further to think about related to the current topic, and encourages self-reflection of strengths and areas needing improvement. Writing exercises need be only a paragraph or two in length and require only minutes of time to complete (Angelo & Cross, 1993; Cross & Angelo, 1988). In the case example (Table 4.1), students are asked to respond by reacting individually to a physician's inappropriate comment, "lots of kids bleed, don't worry about it." This reflective prompt stems from the focused question in paragraph 2 (see Table 4.1), when the student is asked: "What course of action is indicated if an abnormal finding occurs?" The logical answer is to apply pressure to prevent hemorrhage and call the physician to report the finding. The added dimension of an inappropriate physician response stimulates the student to consider individually the options, actions, and consequences with yet another dilemma complicating the situation.

As in the first "Unfolding Case" example, Table 4.2 highlights another specific physiological problem that can be covered using

TABLE 4.2 **Unfolding Case Example Including Possible Answers with a Spinal Cord Injury Scenario**

Learning Outcomes

1. List priorities of care at the scene of the accident.
2. List the main cause of respiratory distress in the spinal cord-injured patient.
3. Recognize appropriate interventions as the client changes over the course of injury and rehabilitation.
4. Verbalize potential or actual nursing problems related to the data in the case.
5. Recognize signs of impending collaborative problems and intervene appropriately.

Paragraph 1

Kerry Fisher, a 19-year-old college sophomore, is involved in a head-on collision. At the scene of the accident, you find Kerry sitting in the front driver's seat. You note the windshield is broken in a large star pattern directly over the steering wheel. Kerry is unconscious.

Focused Questions and Cooperative-Learning Strategies

What would your priorities be? **Roundtable**

Possible answers:

1. Assess and establish an airway if needed using jaw-thrust; assess for bleeding/circulation problems.
2. Immobilize head/neck; do not move him—potential for spinal cord injury.
3. Assess for other injuries—head or internal injury.

Paragraph 2

Kerry develops shallow breathing with periods of apnea en route to the hospital. The hospital is 3 minutes away, and the rescue team decides to administer oxygen with an Ambu bag.

Focused Questions and Cooperative-Learning Strategies

What is the main cause of respiratory distress in a spinal cord-injured patient? **Think-Pair-Share**

Possible answer:
Spinal shock.

(continued)

TABLE 4.2 *(continued)*

Paragraph 3

On admission to the ER, BP is 80/40, p 42, R12, T 95, bowel sounds are absent, and bladder is distended. He is unconscious, and breathing is irregular.

Focused Questions and Cooperative-Learning Strategies

What interventions do you anticipate?   **Roundtable/Pass the Problem**

Possible answers:
Assess and manage respiratory distress; ABGs, intubate, O_2, Swanz and cardiac monitoring; vasopressors for BP and p; NG tube, Foley catheter, methyprednisolone (Medrol) for cord edema; x-rays, MRI, later EMG to assess level of injury.

Paragraph 4

Kerry is past the spinal shock, and neurogenic response is under control. His spine is stabilized with cervical traction, and he is placed on a Stryker frame. An initial home visit to assess Kerry's access to his home reveals several concrete stairs to all entrances. His mother indicates that there are no available funds to construct a ramp.

Focused Questions and Cooperative-Learning Strategies

What nursing problems do you anticipate as healing occurs?   **Think-Pair-Share**

Possible answers:

1. Impaired physical mobility (skin-turn, pin care, massage bony prominences-decubiti)
2. Impaired gas exchange/ineffective breathing patterns—level of injury will impede breathing; need help with cough; deep breathing; suctioning—limit as bradycardia
3. Elimination—self-cath, reflex voiding; suppository/timing
4. Sexual dysfunction
5. Self-esteem
6. Potential infection (pins, UTI, URI)
7. Potential impaired skin integrity (decubiti)
8. Impaired home maintenance; lack of finances to construct home for wheelchair

TABLE 4.2   *(continued)*

Paragraph 5

Kerry's Foley catheter was removed 6 hours ago. When you assessed him 30 minutes ago, he was lying in bed talking to his parents. VS, p 96, 120/60, R20, T98.3. Kerry complained of a severe pounding headache. You repeat his VS and find p50, 180/110, R28, T98.5. You notice goose bumps on his arms.

Focused Questions and Cooperative-Learning Strategies

What is happening to Kerry?   **Think-Pair-Share**
What is your first response?
What do you assess to correct the problem?
What medications will treat the problem?

Possible answers:
Autonomic dysreflexia; hyperreflexia
Raise the head of the bed
Assess bladder, insert Foley; assess rectum for impaction; and assess skin for burns
Apresoline and nifedipine

Reflective-Writing Prompt

Kerry's girlfriend, Anna, has visited Kerry throughout the hospitalization, but her visits have become more infrequent during rehabilitation. Kerry is becoming increasingly concerned and depressed over the situation. Write your feelings from Anna's perspective and Kerry's perspective. Does the nurse have a role in this situation?

---

an interactive format. The five paragraphs of this case follow Kerry, a spinal cord-injured client, from the scene of the accident to the emergency room through hospitalization and rehabilitation. Through the use of cooperative-learning strategies, groups of students process focused questions related to the desired learning outcomes expected by the faculty member (see Table 4.2). The reflective-writing prompt changes the focus of the case from one of dealing with physiological data to the emotional components.

Table 4.3 gives another "Unfolding Case" example dealing with a chemically dependent peer. Staff development educators as well as nurse educators could use this case for their staff or students to process solutions to this common problem. This three-paragraph case requires participants to examine issues related to this situation before actually experiencing it. It is hoped that this

TABLE 4.3   Case Example for Staff Development

Learning Outcomes

After processing the case, the nurse will be able to

- Describe possible solutions to dealing with an alcohol dependent peer.
- Identify ethical and legal conflicts faced when dealing with an alcohol dependent peer.

Paragraph 1

Nancy Nurse works on a surgical unit full-time evenings. She often works with Susan Nurse, who floats between evenings and nights. The last two evenings Nancy has noticed drastic changes in Susan's appearance and work habits. Susan has come to work appearing very sloppy in appearance—wrinkled uniform, runs in her hose, and mussed hair. She always seemed to be "finished" with her work and spent a lot of time in the lounge smoking. Nancy had noticed this behavior and was beginning to worry about Susan's patients.

Focused Questions and Cooperative-Learning Strategies

Group 1	What could be happening?	**Roundtable**
Group 2	What information do you need that you don't have?	**Roundtable**
Group 3	What should Nancy do?	**Roundtable** After all three groups finish processing, they "pass the problem" to a new group and that group adds to and clarifies the list. Then, another group "passes the problem." This time, the new group circles the best or most probable answers. Each group reports.

Paragraph 2

Nancy and Susan work together again. This time, Susan repeats her prior actions, but this time Nancy smells a distinctive alcoholic odor on her breath. She also notices that Susan seems shaky and unstable. Nancy asks Susan if she is OK and offers to call the supervisor for her so she could go home sick. Susan refuses, saying she cannot leave because she needs the hours and that she is just tired from "partying" last night. She promises that if Nancy does not expose her for coming to work "a little high" she'll never do it again.

TABLE 4.3   *(continued)*

Focused Questions and Cooperative-Learning Strategies

Pairs of students	What should Nancy do?	**Think-Pair-Share, then**
	What is the ethical dilemma?	**Pairs report.**
	What are her alternatives and possible consequences of each?	

Paragraph 3

Nancy works with Susan again, and the behavior repeats itself. She also catches Nancy "spiking" her coffee with a flask of "Southern Comfort" she conveniently keeps in her purse. Nancy confronts her and asks her to seek help through employee health. She refuses, so Nancy confides and seeks help from another staff nurse, Heather. Heather tells Nancy to mind her own business. She tells her that because she is married, she does not understand how important it is to a single person like Susan to "party" and try to find a man and a father for her 2-year-old son. She also tells Nancy to suggest to Susan to use mouthwash so no one else notices.

Focused Questions and Cooperative-Learning Strategies

Why does Heather ignore and rationalize the situation? Considering all the data, what should Nancy do?   **Roundtable and group reporting.**

Reflective-Writing Prompt

How would you feel about working with a recovered chemically dependent nurse?

exercise will stimulate discussion related to the proper procedures that need to be followed for them to fulfill their professional responsibility, protect clients, and help chemically dependent co-workers. The reflective-writing prompt stimulates the nurse to examine personal values and beliefs related to a recovered peer. Again, processing one's feelings and thoughts about an issue before experiencing it helps the nurse function more effectively when actually faced with the situation.

"Unfolding Cases" is a comprehensive teaching plan that allows educators to promote critical thinking, communication skills, and active involvement while also promoting continuous improvement through self-reflection. Using this design, professors and staff development educators can create cases to meet specific learning outcomes, allowing students or staff nurses to be immersed in situations dealing with multifaceted data. Students come away from this experience with a sense of being able to solve complex problems with a variety of new and creative solutions. Their self-confidence is enhanced as is their ability to deal effectively with the challenges nurses face in practice. This method is diverse and its flexibility meets varied learning outcomes. It can be used as a classroom activity, a homework activity to prepare for class, a post-conference activity, or as a make-up for a missed clinical day. Glendon and Ulrich's (2001) workbook of "Unfolding Cases" across the nursing curriculum highlights a variety of cases that are ready to be implemented by nursing faculty.

UNFOLDING FAMILY CASES

Unfolding Family Cases is a variation of "Unfolding Cases." The elements of the case remain the same as in the unfolding case (purpose, biographical data, context, and content), but the case unfolds across the course or curriculum rather than a single class. It focuses on the individual client and the impact the problem has on the client's family. It provides for multiple branching of concepts or specific problems rather than a static predetermined sequence of events, which is the norm with "Unfolding Cases."

In developing an "Unfolding Family Case," the faculty member creates five fictional families (see Table 4.4). Students are divided into groups of five to form "primary groups." The total number of groups will depend on the number of students in the class. For example, if there are 40 students, 8 groups will be formed. Each group member is assigned a different fictional family to work with throughout the course. Periodically, "wild cards" are introduced, and students reflect in writing and discuss in groups the characteristics of the "wild card" and the impact this specific "wild card" might have on the family with which they are working.

TABLE 4.4   Fictional Family Examples

1   Amy Bryant is a 16-year-old Appalachian single female. She lives with her parents and six younger siblings in the "hills" of Beaver, Ohio. She attends 9th grade and has a 16-year-old boyfriend. Her family is on public assistance. She has just discovered that she is pregnant.

2   John and Irene Wong are Chinese immigrants who have recently come to the United States. They are both in their early 20s. They live in a small one-bedroom apartment above a Chinese restaurant in downtown Chicago. Both of them work at the restaurant in exchange for the apartment and a small salary. They are expecting their first child.

3   Kate McCoy and Alice Robbins are a lesbian couple who have a long-term relationship of 5 years. Kate is 38 years old and is a college Spanish professor. Alice is 42, never been married, and working as a criminal lawyer. She has hypertension and diabetes. The couple has decided to have a child together, and Kate has just found out that the artificial insemination with donor sperm has resulted in pregnancy.

4   Sarah and Jake Mullins, 44 and 48, respectively, have been married for 15 years and have had infertility problems. After trying for 10 years to become pregnant, they decided to accept the fact that they would have no children. They are financially comfortable, and both have full-time jobs, Sarah as an office manager and Jake as a marketing executive. Sarah has just found out she is pregnant.

5   Tara Cristoff is 26 years old. She has a 3-year-old son and has just gotten divorced after her husband of 4 years walked out on her. She had a one-night stand, and now she is pregnant. She is unsure if the father of the baby is the one-night stand or her ex-husband. She is getting child support but has no job at the present. She is very depressed and is afraid to tell her ex-husband that she is pregnant. Her mother lives 450 miles away and is unaware of the pregnancy or divorce.

In creating fictional families, the faculty member needs to include a variety of elements, such as culture, age, marital status, family composition, educational background, socioeconomic status, and content relevant to the objectives of the course. Table 4.4 gives an example of five such families used to teach a basic obstetrical course. It is important to create five very different families to increase the learning and broaden the scope of discussion among students.

"Wild cards" are potential situation-specific, developmental crises or common problems that might occur in the situation created within the families. Students, in their primary groups, choose one of five cards, each depicting a different type of problem to be integrated into their fictional family. "Wild cards" are introduced periodically in the course, as new content might be in a traditional course. Figure 4.1 shows an example of how this process might proceed for one student throughout the course. This particular student selected family 1, Amy's family, to work on throughout the course. The first group of "wild cards" introduced were five potential scenarios that could occur during the first trimester of pregnancy. Note that in Figure 4.1, "normal" is used as one possible scenario as well as the problematic ones. The second set of "wild cards" presents problems of second and third trimester, and the third set of problems during labor and delivery. At selected intervals, the student would choose one of the five cards to integrate into her or his family. "Wild cards" are always drawn while students are in their "primary group" to assure a wider variance of different problems for different families. In this particular case, the student might choose "threatened abortion" first, then "pregnancy induced hypertension" (PIH), and then "premature labor." A unique sequence of problems would be integrated into family 1 through this student's contributions to the group and class discussion. How the case evolves for each student will be different and will depend on the cards they draw. This will create a multitude of variations, which will make for better and varied discussion in the class.

After each set of "wild cards" is drawn, students are given work to complete outside of class, on an individual basis, related to both

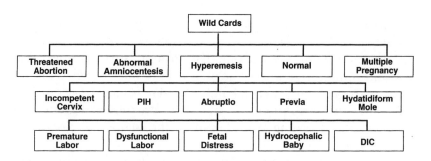

FIGURE 4.1 Amy's case unfolding.

the "problem" and the effect it may have on their family. This work is in the form of a two-part study guide asking for pertinent information on the "problem" in the first part, and a few open-ended questions to stimulate thinking as to how their particular family might react in the second part (see Table 4.5). This information is to be recorded and reflected on in writing for use in the next class.

At the next class students are grouped into "wild card groups" or groups comprising all students who have selected the same "wild card" but have different families. For example, all student selecting "threatened abortion" will group together. In this particular case, there will always be five different groups because there are only five different "wild cards." Yet the number of students in each group will vary, depending on the number of students in the class. If there are 40 students in the class, there will be five groups of eight each. In these "wild card" groups, they first discuss part one

TABLE 4.5   Study Guide

Part 1

1. Define the problem or condition.
2. Describe the common signs and symptoms of the problem or condition.
3. Discuss normal/abnormal laboratory data or testing needed to evaluate or diagnose.
4. Describe the usual treatment regime.
5. Describe nursing interventions appropriate in this case.
6. List possible and the most probable client outcome(s).

Part 2

1. How will your "wild card" affect your family in the following areas?

    • Feelings and reactions of family members and client (coping)
    • Communication among family members
    • Power and decision making in the family
    • Cultural implications
    • Resources and support systems
    • Potential ethical and legal dilemmas

2. What are the strengths and areas needing support in this family?

of the study guide and come up with a group version of answers based on the discussion and input of all students. Then the groups, using *Roundtable* (see Chapter 3), answer and discuss a set of focused questions prepared by the faculty member (see Table 4.6). A total class discussion follows as each group presents the "wild card" including answers to part 1 of the study guide and focused questions. Through class discussion, students are exposed to information on all five "wild card" problems, not just the one they drew. At this time, the faculty member can summarize important concepts, clarify and correct misconceptions, and answer questions as they arise. Important information and content are covered, but the faculty members take on the role of facilitators rather than the traditional role of experts. The student group that researched the specific topic becomes the ones responsible for helping other students in the class learn and comprehend the material.

The next phase of the model regroups the class into "family functioning" groups of students who selected the same family initially. These groups comprise students who have the same family but different "wild cards." Again, there will be five groups because there are five families, but the number of students in each group will vary according to the number in the class. In these groups, students using Roundtable (see Chapter 3) process another group of focused questions related to family issues dealing with the selected "wild card" problems. These are identical to the ones listed in part 2 of the study guide (see Table 4.5). Once again, a total class discussion follows as each group reports its findings to the class.

Figure 4.2 visually depicts the entire process of Unfolding Family Cases. This process can be used as the basis for an entire course, as shown in this example, or as a part of a course. It has great versatility in that it can be adapted to any content area. If a

TABLE 4.6 Wild Card Group-Focused Questions

1. What are the similarities and differences in the way your family most likely reacted to this wild card problem/condition?
2. What factors contributed to the differences or similarities (culture, family composition, financial status, age, etc.)?

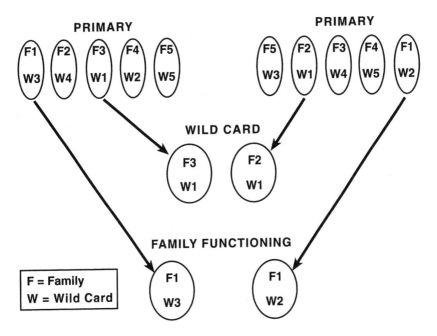

FIGURE 4.2   Student grouping for unfolding family cases.

family development course is being taught, the "wild cards" could be family crises or common problems families encounter as they develop. It meets requirements of the new learning paradigm in that it results in students being able to think critically, interact with others, and practice social and presentation skills. It is a vehicle that allows faculty to cover the content, yet keep students involved and interactive in the process. It also turns factual content into real-life situations and allows students to learn to solve problems of application in a safe and stimulating environment.

Again, the previous examples of "Unfolding Cases" and "Unfolding Family Cases" showed how the Comprehensive Group-Learning Model can be used in its entirety, but pieces or parts of it can be used as well. Remember, teachers select strategies that best meet their learning objectives. They can mix, match, combine, and be creative as they put these strategies to use.

CHAPTER 5

Using Experiential Learning Strategies

Faculty can stimulate students holistically through their senses, enhance critical thinking, and involve them in groups at the same time, all of which multiplies the learning potential of students. Students are tapped holistically through vision, hearing, emotions, intellect, and physical dimensions. This chapter discusses a multitude of teaching strategies and learning modalities, which can be used to stimulate memory and enhance the problem-solving abilities of the students.

FACULTY DRAWINGS

Stimulating students through the use of their senses is a good way to promote learning of common signs and symptoms related to various disease states. Recognizing distinguishing characteristics of specific client's problems is a primary role of the nurse. Artwork is a unique way to bring these signs and symptoms to life and help nurses remember the many distinct clinical signs associated with a client's disease. Drawings of a client can slightly exaggerate the clinical characterizations in a way textbook photographs do not depict them, which helps trigger the student's memory. Critical thinking related to this material can be accomplished by using specific focused questions created by the teacher to stimulate students intellectually. Questions can be formulated that encourage student analysis of the data in the artwork, or more complex questions can stimulate student problem solving. This group strategy combines the use of art work and focused questions to encourage students to apply knowledge related to a particular disease state.

Students view the picture while sitting together in a circle. After viewing the picture in detail, students, in a group, answer the questions that are found typed below the artwork. For example, Figure 5.1, a patient with Graves' disease, might be shown to the student group. After viewing the drawing, the students are asked to respond to the focused questions below it. Initially, the questions should focus on the clinical manifestations shown in the drawing as well as challenge students to add additional data by labeling

Focused Questions:
What are the clinical manifestations of Graves' disease?
What are common treatment measures?

diet _____

medications _____

Label other pertinent signs on the drawing that are descriptive of Graves disease.

Pick 3 nursing problems and describe the nursing care.

FIGURE 5.1   Drawing of a client with Graves' disease.

common characteristics not addressed in the drawing. In this example, diarrhea, tachycardia, insomnia, and rapid speech are clinical signs not easily depicted in a drawing, whereas goiter, exophthalmos, and heat intolerance are physical signs that are apparent in the artwork. Nursing problems and their subsequent interventions require in-depth analysis of the data. In their group, students are then required to select three problems related to the client depicted in the artwork, and then discuss and plan nursing interventions for this client, including actual and potential problems. Once individual groups have answered all of the focused questions and designed a plan of care, a group representative shares the answers with the entire class. In this example, students might choose sleep pattern disturbance, body image disturbance, and potential for injury related to corneal injury. Students would present nursing interventions pertinent to these diagnoses. A comprehensive plan of care for the client would evolve as all groups presented their chosen nursing problems and interventions.

Artwork serves to stimulate the students' senses and encourages memory of the clinical signs. Focused questions help students use critical thinking skills to process the information by analyzing the data and determining appropriate nursing diagnoses and their interventions. Students could further be challenged by including questions that require them to establish priority or compare and contrast nursing interventions. Combining the two strategies of artwork and focused questions encourages students to remember data as well as synthesize critical questions related to specific disease states.

STUDENT DRAWINGS

Having students draw their clients is a strategy to help them understand the pathophysiology and related signs and symptoms their client is exhibiting. Students are instructed to draw their client including disease pathophysiology, signs and symptoms, medication actions, and even client statements (see Figure 5.2 for an example). It is important to tell them that the drawing technique is not what is important, but it is the content and application that

FIGURE 5.2   Student drawing of client with pregnancy induced hypertension.

you are interested in. They should be creative in their interpretations by using colored pencils or markers, arrows, boxes, an so forth to illustrate their points. These drawings can be done at home as preparation for client care, on the spot in a post-conference activity, or during the clinical day as time permits. After students complete their individual drawings, it is essential for them to share and explain them in a group activity. Group members can suggest ways to augment the drawings through this interaction. The faculty can extend the learning by asking the group Socratic-type focused questions related to the drawings. It is important that faculty praise the drawings for what was done well and ignore the negative aspects, as students are often sensitive about their artistic ability. This activity ensures that all group members increase their understanding of the interconnections between pathophysiology and the nursing interventions critical to client care. Trausch (2003) used the drawing technique with 52 BSN students and found that 90% felt that the time spent on drawings as a clinical preparation was worthwhile whereas only 3% did not. Students commented that drawings increased their comprehension and their ability to retain information. They reported that they could "see where pleural effusion was . . . reading it didn't help," and "this makes things stick in my mind." This exemplifies the theory that experiential activities increase students' ability to discover the connections of things (Dewey, 1944).

CONCEPT JIGSAW

Another way to use artwork and stimulate critical thinking is to combine student artwork with the cooperative-learning strategy Jigsaw (Aronson et al., 1978). The *Concept Jigsaw* is a group strategy that helps students investigate a variety of topics within a complex concept. It is a strategy that helps the professor cover and process a variety of related topics in an organized and efficient manner. This strategy combines the basic steps of Jigsaw (see Table 3.1) and group artwork. Individual members of each student group are given different pieces of an overall concept so that within each group the total is examined in detail. Students are given study guides to direct their research into their topic and to assure that the common themes are identified and investigated. They are also asked to depict their piece of the concept visually. After individual work is completed, students come together in their group. As a group, they discuss their part, show their individual visual depictions, and become "experts" on the total topic assigned. At this point, from each individual's artwork and completed study guides, the group is asked to depict visually and label the assigned topic in a creative way that illustrates its main features. Students are stimulated intellectually to remember things better when they can not only visualize but actually physically create the depiction of important aspects of the topic. Students then regroup so that there is an "expert" on each part of each group (see Figure 3.4). In their new groups, students present their group's drawing as they explain their part, in turn, to one another. As a result, all students have been exposed to the total concept and have visualized the similarities and differences within a common group of topics. A teacher-led total class discussion completes the strategy.

For example, this strategy is an excellent way of teaching students about growth and development throughout the life span, while encouraging critical thinking about the characteristics, similarities, and differences in stages. Students are assigned to groups of five. Each group is assigned a specific developmental stage, such as infancy, toddlerhood, preschooler, school-ager, and adolescence. Within each group, individual members are assigned five different areas to research—physical characteristics, cognitive abilities, psychosocial aspects, spiritual and moral development, and health promotion and prevention needs. Individual students are given a study guide to direct them in identifying the major themes important to examine within their area. For example, the student who was assigned health promotion and prevention needs of the infant might be asked to identify the immunizations necessary for the first year of life (see Table 5.1). At the next class, students get together within their initial groups and teach their part to the rest of the group, so that this group is knowledgeable about all aspects of infancy. At this point, students, as a group, draw and label their idea of that particular developmental stage. For example, students in the infant group might draw an infant with a large head, flexed posture, fontanels, and immunizations listed with an arrow directed toward the thigh (see Figure 5.3). Students then regroup so that an "expert" on each developmental stage is in each group. "Experts" explain, discuss, and share their artwork on their assigned developmental stage. At this point, each student has been exposed to every developmental stage and is better prepared for the overall class discussion that follows. The teacher then leads an overall discussion of each developmental stage as groups share their artwork and explain the rationale for their visual depictions. This is an excellent time to discuss variations within normal development and possible stereotypical thinking.

TABLE 5.1   Infancy—Study Guide for Concept Jigsaw

Physical	1.	List characteristics about weight at 6 and 12 months.
	2.	When do they roll over, sit up, crawl, walk?
	3.	Describe eating patterns.
	4.	Describe elimination patterns.
Cognitive	1.	Describe the outcomes of the sensorimotor period.
	2.	What is object permiance, and when is it likely to occur?
	3.	Describe the relationship between crying and infant language development.
Psychosocial	1.	When do they smile?
	2.	What are development tasks related to Erikson?
	3.	What are the characteristics of bonding?
	4.	Describe separation anxiety, and when it is likely to occur.
Spiritual-moral	1.	Give some examples of rituals specific to infancy.
Health promotion/ prevention	1.	What immunizations are required during the first year?
	2.	What would you tell a mother about safety for this period of development?
	3.	What play activities/toys would you suggest for infant development?

This strategy can also be used to discuss leadership styles, different modes of delivering nursing care, or concepts of teaching and learning. The possibilities are endless. Again, it is an excellent way to cover broad concepts quickly yet thoroughly, while actively involving students—a key to improving learning.

PHOTOGRAPHS

The use of photographs and focused questions can be employed in much the same way as drawings. However, with a photograph, a real client can be used as a basis for a specific learning outcome. Similarly, focused questions can trigger problem-solving methods of students. For example, students may be shown a photograph of a client with cirrhosis of the liver. In this photograph, students could recognize the classic signs and symptoms, such as jaundice, massive ascites, everted umbilicus, dilated upper abdominal veins,

FIGURE 5.3   Example of artwork for infancy period in Concept Jigsaw.

and ankle edema. An initial focused question might ask, "What are the classic signs of liver disease?" Answers could include the obvious ones from the photograph or others, such as pruritus, vomiting, clay-colored stools, and coke-colored urine. A second more detailed and specific question could ask the students to cite the clinical signs specific to cirrhosis and how it differs from a patient with hepatitis A. A third question might stimulate students to explain the life-threatening complications pertaining to cirrhosis of the liver or challenge students to analyze and choose a priority nursing intervention from data given to them by faculty. With cirrhosis of the liver, students should be able to identify a potential for hemorrhage related to esophageal varices from clinical data given about the patient's hematemesis, rapid heart rate (110), and decreased blood pressure (80/40). In a fourth variation, the teacher might also give data on two patients with liver disease, one with hepatitis A and one with cirrhosis. Students could be asked not only to compare the signs and symptoms of these liver diseases but also to analyze the differences in treatment modalities. For example, students should be able to recognize that the diet of a client with hepatitis would include protein, whereas the diet for a client with advanced cirrhosis complicated by portal system encephalopathy would require limiting the protein intake. Again, once individual groups have processed the focused questions, they share results with the entire class. At this point, a total class discussion evolves.

VIDEO, FILMS, AND TELEVISION

Video is yet another way to stimulate the senses; video adds the hearing and kinesthetic dimensions missing in artwork and photographs. Students see, hear, and watch interactions, which makes the learning situation feel the most real in comparison with artwork or photographs. Video can be designed in such a way by the faculty to portray a certain message, and the information can be tailored or staged to fit students' learning needs. If video production is too time-consuming, an alternative method of using video segments from existing commercial videotapes, feature films, or television shows can be just as effective and easy to accomplish. Focused questions are added at the designated moments in the chosen video medium and provide the framework for student problem solving and analysis. Student groups may be challenged to view the tape and answer faculty-posed questions either at the end of the tape or at various intervals throughout the tape. Faculty can stimulate communication-related or action-oriented responses to questions. For example, "What do you think is an appropriate response or action by the nurse given the situation just viewed?" Students report their ideas, and class discussion ensues. At that point, the next segment of the video demonstrates either what the nurse said or did, or both. Students see the results of the nurse's interventions and proceed with additional processing of the current situation. Different segments can be used to process pathophysiology, pertinent nursing interventions, and communication with patients or other health team members. For example, in a faculty-produced video, a scenario of the nurse who is confronted with the client experiencing low blood sugar may be presented. The actor, as a patient, demonstrates the classic symptoms of low blood sugar—anxiety, shaking, and headache. The segment is stopped, and the instructor asks, "What could be going on with this client?" and "What should be done immediately?" At this point, groups analyze the information provided and share their analysis and solutions. The next segment of the video is shown, and the students observe that the client indeed has a low blood sugar as verified by the result of an Accucheck, and the client is given 4 ounces of orange juice. Students get immediate feedback on the appropriateness of their group's analysis and solutions. Other segments could follow with questions focusing on what could happen if treatment were not obtained or if treatment did not help, or what are other alternative interventions.

One particularly excellent classic videotape, *Don't Cry For Me* (Gandolfi, Tringali, & Cole, 1985), is a film highlighting the lives of adolescents with cystic fibrosis (CF). This film vividly shows the physical appearance of several different adolescents and examples of their daily regimes. Several adolescents discuss their thoughts and feelings about having CF. The teacher stops the video at various intervals and asks groups to answer pertinent focused questions regarding the segment. The learning is compounded by tapping students holistically through viewing and hearing the segments and the critical thinking required of the focused questions. Two other excellent films are *Living With AIDS* (DiFeliciantonio, 1986), a film about a young, white, homosexual man, and *Special Care* (Centre Productions, 1984), a film about children born prematurely and their diverse experiences in the neonatal intensive care unit. Faculty could also use television series or feature films to help students evaluate family-processing or cultural differences. In groups, students view several episodes of a particular show or an entire feature film and complete a family assessment and care plan based on family theory. For example, students might view *Roseanne*, *Grace Under Fire*, or the film *Parenthood* as the basis for the process (Ulrich, Teets, & Quinn, 1994). Students could also analyze a *Star Trek* episode depicting communication patterns, cultural norms, and interactional patterns associated with characters from the different planets. After viewing the episode, students, in groups, could be asked to respond to focused questions, such as, "Were the communities of these two different cultures competitive or cooperative?" and "How were the communication patterns of the two cultures similar or different?" In this way, students can vividly recognize these differences that will help them recognize subtler differences in existing cultures. The popular film *My Life* can be used in a family health systems course. Students can follow the life of a young man diagnosed with cancer at the time his wife becomes pregnant. His goal becomes a task of leaving his unborn son a "handbook of life." The film's characters exemplify common coping mechanisms, dysfunctional communication, and spirituality as they face a crisis in their lives. Students are able to apply important concepts as they follow the life of this couple (Parker & Faulk, 2004). Short clips from cable television show such as *The Baby Story*, *Labor and Delivery*, *ER*, and so forth, can be invaluable in making a point during a classroom presentation.

SIMULATION

Simulation is another way to stimulate the senses and evoke critical thinking. Student pairs could be asked to view a typical simulated hospital room. The room would have a client sleeping in a hospital bed and would be set up to mock several safety hazards. These hazards might include such things as the Foley bag touching the floor, uncapped syringes lying at the bedside, the bed in high position, and side rails down. When asked, "What's wrong with this scene?" each student pair will generate a list of the problems they identify. The total class then reconvenes, and each pair shares the findings as the instructor records the hazards on the board. As each hazard is identified, the instructor discusses the significance of the hazard and encourages student pairs to think of ways to prevent the hazard from occurring. Other ways to extend the learning are for faculty to propose focused questions that challenge students to think of ways to manage these breaks in safety standards.

Variations of this strategy might include having the students imagine the client in a different developmental stage, such as a child or an elderly person. Critical thinking is enhanced further by adding information and changing the focused questions to things such as, "What is missing in the mock scene?" or "What is the first thing the nurse should do when he or she enters the room?" Faculty could also insert additional information about the client, such as laboratory results, or recent nurses' notes, to make the situation more complex and extend the critical thinking process. For example, a sample scenario of a child with a tonsillectomy could challenge the students to study the environment and identify the need for the Yanker suction equipment at the bedside. Setting up a mock code situation (Spunt, Foster, & Adams, 2004) or a typical hospital room to help a new student learn how to begin care (Ham & O'Rourke, 2004) are other ideas using simulation. Also the use of the new "Sim Man," a computerized patient model, can simulate a variety of clinical situations in which students can practice their critical thinking skills (Feingold, Calaluce, & Kallen, 2004). Simulations create a sense of reality yet allow faculty to encourage problem solving without the risk of client injury.

Simulation is a good way to ensure student's comprehension of the principles involved in dressing changes, catheter insertion, intravenous administration, medication administration, and other skill-related tasks involved in the nursing role. Faculty can demonstrate the skill involved incorrectly in front of a group of students. The group is challenged to critique and list all the breaks in technique on the board or overhead. After the demonstration, the group members are asked to list all of the principles that must be followed while performing the skill they just observed. Then, using the list of errors, they identify which principles were violated by the faculty member. Two benefits of this technique are that the faculty member makes the errors instead of the student, which puts students more at ease in their novice state, and that it encourages them to use critical thinking about the principles involved in the skill rather than memorizing a step-by-step approach to learning the nursing task.

EMPATHY EXPERIENCES

Empathy experiences connect students' feelings and emotions related to the patient and the situation and stimulates a deeper learning. Faculty tap the students' emotions in these experiences and stimulate them to imagine the perspective of another person.

Nurses are called upon to care for individuals with problems and life experiences that are often vastly different from their own. Planning experiences that build insight into the patient's unique needs helps the student to move from feeling only sympathy for the patient to having empathy or understanding. Ultimately, this understanding leads the nurse to help the patient set realistic goals. Activities that put the student nurse into the position of feeling what it is like to be ill, homeless, disabled, or different from others kindles the development of insight into the patient's needs and begins to instill a foundation for caring, which is essential to nursing practice.

There are several commonly used ways to place students in this unique position and help them get a glimpse of what it might feel like to be a patient. Student groups are assigned to explore an empathy experience. Students choose to pretend to be a diabetic for a day by following a prescribed diet and sticking themselves for blood sugars, spend a day in a wheelchair, or wear socks over their hands to simulate a physical disability. It also may require them to perform activities like eating, writing, or buttoning their clothes while simulating the disability. Placing students in pairs works best for this experience. One student experiences the activity, and the other student observes or takes on the role of frustrating the other student with obstacles or negative comments, such as, "hurry up, we're late." In contrast, the observer could also take the role of helping the student patient feel accepted. Students should be cautioned that this is a pretend activity, and safety precautions must be taken as indicated by the activity. Students could be given the choice of this activity or another assignment. In other words, the student volunteers to participate, as developing caring requires a desire by the student to truly experience this feeling state. Other activities that could be substituted are interviewing or spending the day with someone who is disabled, chronically ill, or wheelchair bound.

Once each student pair has completed the experience, the pair returns to the group. The entire group shares its experiences with each other and decides on a way to present ideas, experiences, and insights to the whole class. For example, this could be accomplished with a paper, poster, presentation, poem, quilt, or other artistic expressions. In this way, students are exposed to a variety of feeling states through the eyes of others.

FISH BONE

The *Fish Bone* strategy (Ishikawa, 1982) is a cognitive problem-solving structure that has frequently been used in the business field and is easily adapted to the educational setting. It is a useful technique that educators can use to stimulate critical thinking among students and at the same time promote the concepts of teamwork and cooperation, skills essential in professional nursing. Learning this strategy is especially beneficial because as practicing nurses, students will be expected to use this problem-solving method when they are members of continuous quality improvement teams, a concept popular and pervasive in the work world.

To apply the Fish Bone strategy, faculty members assign students to heterogeneous groups of four to five members. The professor poses a problem and the groups must identify the potential cause of this problem, using the Fish Bone diagram (see Figure 5.4), which illustrates a cause-and-effect relationship. The groups brainstorm a list of potential causes for the problem. Ishikawa (1982), the original creator of Fish Bone, used four general areas under which to categorize the causes in order to stimulate the group's brainstorming: people, methods, material/supplies, and equipment. Categories are meant to prompt student thinking, not limit the brainstorming process. If desired, the professor can eliminate the categories to encourage the free flow of ideas. There are several ways to record the group's ideas. As ideas are generated, the blackboard in the classroom could be used, or students could

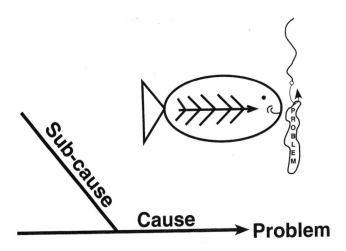

FIGURE 5.4   Fish Bone diagram. From Ulrich, D., & Glendon, K. (1994). Fishbone strategy: A TQM strategy applied to nursing education. *Nurse Educator, 19,* 7–8. Reprinted with permission.

use a pad of paper on which to draw the Fish Bone and record the information in turn. Another especially useful tool is the use of "Post-It Notes" to record ideas. These are good to use because they can easily be moved around on the diagram, which is important when combining the like causes, the next step in the process. Students often contribute the same idea, although perhaps in different words, so identical causes can be combined, and the group can come up with one "Post-It," incorporating all similar ideas for the Fish Bone. Brainstorming should not be stopped to settle these issues, but collated in the second step of the process, after brainstorming is complete.

As described by Ulrich and Glendon (1994), the professor could pose the problem that "the number of people contracting the AIDS virus continues to increase, despite an increased awareness of the disease." In completing the diagram, under the category of "people" (if categories are being used), students might list "unsafe sex practices continue to exist" as a cause of the problem. If individual students report a similar idea, then these are clarified and combined in the second step by asking these students if their idea has a uniquely different meaning. After causes are determined, students must be encouraged to include sub-causes on the diagram. Sub-causes often lead to uncovering the actual root cause of a problem. A way to elicit these sub-causes is to encourage students to ask the "why" question of the cause generated: "Why do unsafe sex practices continue to exist?" In this case, two sub-causes might be "the attitude that people believe they will not contract AIDS or a lack of accurate knowledge regarding the spread of the disease exists." Students should be encouraged to continue to ask the "why" question of these sub-causes until answers are exhausted. Similarly, sub-causes should be investigated with all other causes that were previously generated. Finally, through group consensus, the group circles the potential root cause for further investigation. In this example, students, by consensus, might circle the root cause: "the attitude that people believe they will not contract AIDS." Students would then be encouraged to do further study using objective methods to validate that this is actually the root cause of the problem. To complete this strategy, students would need to collect data to verify the root cause circled. In this case, students might conduct a survey of student attitudes about contracting AIDS. Once the root cause is identified, students could determine appropriate solutions to this societal problem based on facts, not intuition. Instructors can adapt this tool to students' educational needs by interrupting this process at any point to engage students in class discussion or debate. Figure 5.5 summarizes the steps of the Fish Bone strategy.

The Fish Bone is a versatile strategy that can be adapted to many nursing situations with students or staff. Staff nurses could brainstorm a list of problems using the Roundtable technique on their unit, reserving some for study with the Fish Bone strategy. As described by Glendon and Ulrich (1992b), each member of each group writes down on a pad of paper a problem he or she has experienced as the pad is passed from one to another in turn. This ensures that each staff member contributes, and active participation becomes the norm. Common problems that usually surface during this exercise include inequitable assignments, short staffing, quality assurance problems, cost-containment issues, in-

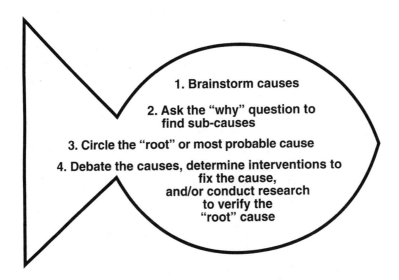

1. Brainstorm causes

2. Ask the "why" question to find sub-causes

3. Circle the "root" or most probable cause

4. Debate the causes, determine interventions to fix the cause, and/or conduct research to verify the "root" cause

FIGURE 5.5   Steps of Fish Bone strategy.

complete shift reports, and patient care dilemmas, to name a few. During this process groups learn and practice social relationship skills that create an environment of acceptance and respect for every member's contribution, which, in turn, increases individual self-esteem and acceptance. Each group then selects one of these identified problems to analyze using Fish Bone. Through the use of a visual fishbone diagram, the groups brainstorm to list potential causes in relation to four general categories on the diagram (people, methods/protocols, materials/supplies, and equipment). These categories help trigger critical thinking related to possible causes. All categories may not be complete, as not every category is germane to every problem. After completing their brainstorming and grouping of like causes, groups, through consensus, circle the most likely root cause for further investigation. For example, a group might choose "inequitable assignments" as a problem. Under the category of "people," staff members might list unequal skill levels of staff as a possible causative factor. Under the category of "methods or unit protocols," group members could list that the charge nurses are the only assignment makers. Inclusion of any potential sub-causes that might exist is critical to the process. One sub-cause of the example—the charge nurse on each shift is the only assignment maker—could be that the charge nurses lack skills in assignment making, or skill levels are inconsistent among charge nurses. A thorough analysis helps the staff to decide the likely root cause on the unit. If the charge nurse is viewed as the main cause of the problem, it is circled on the diagram, and the group's task is complete for this strategy. An additional step of collecting quantitative data is needed to validate this root cause before continuing to the intervention phase. For example, surveying of nurses on all shifts could be done to validate this particular example.

Next, using Pass the Problem (Kagan, 1992), nurses generate interventions to solve the problem based on the identified root cause. The manager collects each group's fish bone and places each one in a separate folder. The folders are then distributed randomly to groups who then decide on possible interventions related to the root cause of each problem. Each folder, complete with interventions, is then passed to another group that adds to and refines the existing list. For example, with the problem of "inequitable assignments," the list of interventions related to the root cause (charge nurse as sole assignment maker) might include rotating choice of assignments, rotating assignment maker, dividing assignment to achieve a balanced patient acuity, choice of keeping assignment for consecutive days, training of charge nurses, or collaborative assignment making. The manager promotes discussion as the interventions are presented and allows staff to reach agreement on interventions to implement. Once the intervention is decided, the manager and staff agree on a period for trial use of the intervention and schedule another team session to evaluate the intervention. When cooperative strategies are used, individual nurses become aware of their importance to the unit. They develop a sense of interdependence and increase their level of personal responsibility to the unit (Aumiller & Rudloff, 1986). This meaningful involvement is an internal motivator that transforms the nurse from a mere worker to a committed, satisfied, and involved member of the organization (see Figure 5.6). Workers who feel ownership, coupled with increased autonomy and responsibility, feel compelled to improve the quality of their performance—in this case, the overall quality of patient care.

FIGURE 5.6 Empowered nurse. From Glendon, K., & Ulrich, D. (1992b). Using cooperative decision making strategies in nursing practice. *Nursing Administration Quarterly,* **17,** 69–73. **Reprinted with permission.**

It is becoming vital that we as nurses learn to analyze problems readily and develop innovative interventions based on factual data. The Fish Bone strategy helps students identify root causes that lead to pinpointing more effective solutions to problems. It connects students cognitively and requires them to think critically and use creative problem-solving techniques.

CONCEPT MAPPING

Dewey recognized early on that learning involved making linkages between what the student already knows and new information (Dewey, 1944). Concept maps take the idea of creating linkages, and as a cognitive structure help students advance their learning. Concept maps borrow all the elements of the nursing process, yet improve upon it by allowing students to visually capture the connections and interrelationships of the whole. In nursing, concept mapping is a visual representation of students' thinking processes as they plan and implement care for their clients. This strategy has also been called mind mapping, clinical thinking web, clinical correlation map, and cognitive maps.

Beitz (1997, 1998) recognized that students needed to be shown a simple concept map to familiarize them with the process and help them gain confidence in their own maps. Figure 5.7 is a simple concept map that could be shared with students as they begin the process of concept mapping. Student maps will need to be produced on large rolls of paper to illustrate the linkages. They may use markers, crayons, colored pencils, and so on, to illustrate their thinking. It is important to emphasize that there are no wrong ways to illustrate concepts and that concept maps may look very different from each other, depending on the depth of understand-

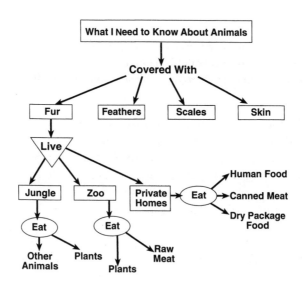

FIGURE 5.7 Simple concept map.

ing the student possesses. Students should be encouraged to be creative. Daley (1996, 1999) realized that clinical practice is an excellent area in which to demonstrate the use of this structure as it helps students visually diagram the process of clinical preparation and what it entails. Recently much has been written about concept mapping and its place in nursing curricula (Mueller, Johnston, & Bligh, 2001; Schuster, 2002). Numerous schools have replaced their nursing care plans with concept maps whereas other schools use the strategy as a post-conference activity or to illustrate concepts in the classroom such as pathophysiology, pharmacology, and so forth. Despite the familiarity of most nursing faculty with the idea of concept maps, it remains a challenge to simplify teaching students how to construct them.

In order to teach students how to develop and use a concept map in clinical practice they must know how to ask the right questions (Table 5.2) and understand the overall process of concept mapping. Figures 5.8–5.14 illustrate one example of the construction of a possible concept map. The example shows only one piece of the map at a time and therefore does not show the layered effect of an actual map because of the space limitation of the authors. Student maps will be much larger, more complicated, and detailed as their creativity and critical thinking blossom.

In Figure 5.8, *What do I look for?*, the basic client information is recorded. In the example shown, the client is a 25-year-old gravida one, para one, first day post-operative cesarean section. Note that the client information is abbreviated and placed within an oval shape and centered on the page. The student may choose to use circles, squares, or triangles to frame the client information. Next, the student is instructed to surround the client information with an organizing framework to facilitate assessment. In this example the functional patterns were used in assessing the client. However, faculty could substitute systems, Maslow's hierarchy of needs, or any other appropriate framework. Note in the example that the pieces of the assessment framework are listed within a box and linked by a line to the client information. Once this information is recorded, students look at each assessment area and pose pertinent questions that will guide their assessment of the client. These questions are recorded adjacent to the box representing the appro-

TABLE 5.2   Asking the Right Questions to Create a Concept Map

What do I look for?

- Create a visual assessment guide based on the information you have been given about your client (name, age, presenting problem, medications).
- Draw boxes that represent each of Gordon's function patterns or another applicable assessment framework such as systems, or Maslow's hierarchy.
- Determine which areas of assessment are essential and list pertinent questions you have in the appropriate functional pattern box for a textbook client matching your client's diagnoses.

What did I find?

- Use this assessment guide to collect assessment data on the client you are caring for.
- Collect data from chart, physical assessment, shift report, etc., related to your client and put it in the appropriate boxes in a new color.
- You may need to add to the functional pattern areas that will individualize your map based on your assigned client.

What's most important?

- Look at the data you collected and determine nursing diagnoses of significance related to the data.
- Write these diagnoses adjacent to the functional pattern and circle them with another color.
- Number each diagnosis as to priority.

What are the connections and interrelationships?

- Look at your map and draw dotted lines connecting diagnoses that influence one another.

What outcomes do I want to achieve?

- List the client-centered outcomes around the nursing diagnoses, connecting them to the diagnoses in a sunburst design.

What interventions do I use?

- For each outcome, list appropriate interventions and connect them with lines to the outcome.

Was my outcome met?

- Evaluate each outcome and state if it was met or not met beside the outcome, listing appropriate data.
- Be creative, use a variety of colors, shapes, dotted lines, bold lines, double lines, or words to connect concepts; there is not correct way to illustrate ideas.

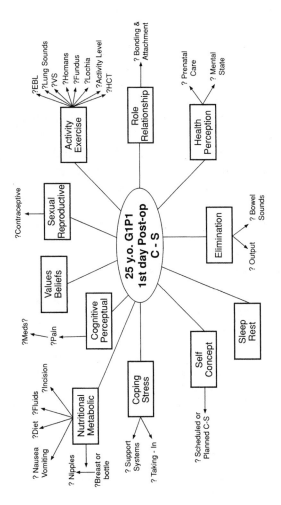

FIGURE 5.8 What do I look for?

priate functional pattern. Note that adjacent to the functional pattern box, Activity Exercise, the questions the student posed were: estimated blood loss (EBL), lung sounds, vital signs, Homans sign, fundus, lochia, activity level, and hematocrit. In preparing for clinical the student should have read about cesearean sections and be cognizant of the potential complications of hemorrhage associated with surgery and postpartum. Each functional pattern is processed in a similar fashion. This initial map is a clinical preparation tool and serves as an assessment guide before the student begins actual assessment of the client.

In Figure 5.9, *What did I find?*, students record in a new color the data found on the chart, from the physical assessment, and shift report, and so on, next to the questions they formulated from the first step. In the example shown the student found a 1000 cc blood loss, clear lung sounds, blood pressure 100/60, pulse 100, respirations 24, and temperature 99F, among other things. If the student finds additional information that was not considered during the preparation phase (Figure 5.8), these data should also be recorded adjacent to the appropriate functional pattern.

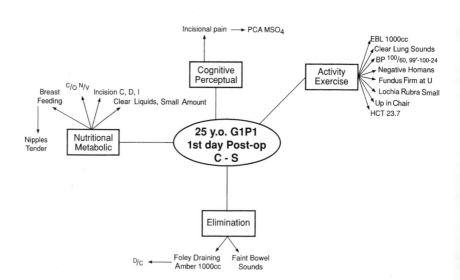

FIGURE 5.9   What did I find?

In Figure 5.10, *What's most important?*, students analyze the assessment data and formulate appropriate nursing diagnoses of significance related to the data. They should write the diagnosis next to the functional pattern and circle them with another color. Then the diagnoses must be numbered as to priority. In this example, five nursing diagnoses were formulated around four of the functional patterns.

In Figure 5.11, *What are the connections?*, the student must draw dotted lines connecting diagnoses that influence one another. In this example, risk for falls is related to pain, ineffective breastfeeding is related to fluid volume deficit, and so on. This step causes the student to look at the client holistically and see the connections and interrelationships of the parts to the whole.

In Figure 5.12, *What outcomes do I want to achieve?*, the student determines client-centered outcomes and centers them around the diagnoses like a sunburst. Note in this figure that one of the outcomes associated with the diagnosis pain is: the client will report

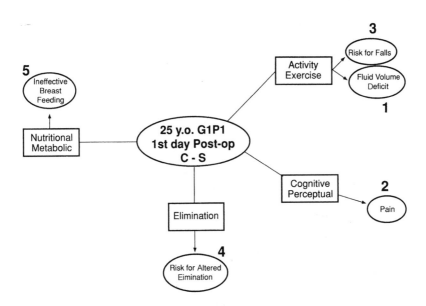

FIGURE 5.10 What's most important?

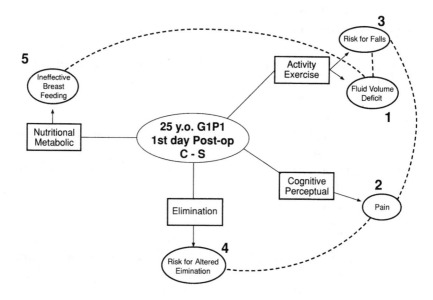

FIGURE 5.11   What are the connections?

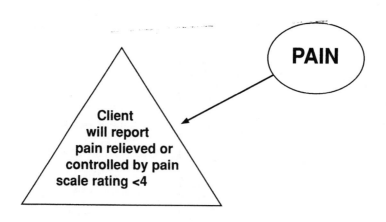

FIGURE 5.12   What outcomes do I want to achieve?

pain relieved or controlled by pain scale rating <4. The student will identify outcomes for each of the diagnoses listed on the map.

In Figure 5.13, *What interventions do I use?*, the student determines interventions for each of the outcomes listed and connects them with lines to the outcome. In this example, one intervention for decreasing the client's pain would be to teach relaxation techniques.

In Figure 5.14, *Was my outcome met?*, the student evaluates each outcome measure post intervention and records next to the outcome whether the outcome was met or not met. In the example, the client outcome was met as she reports a 3 on a pain scale.

Initially, students may fear or feel overwhelmed at the idea of using concept maps. This step-by-step guide will ease their fears and provide structure to a new creative process. The last step in implementing this strategy is to have students share their maps with faculty and each other. By having students develop their own concept maps and then as groups discuss and build upon their

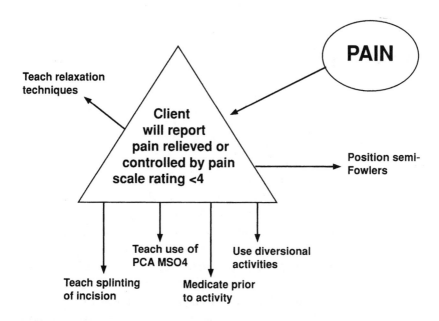

FIGURE 5.13   What interventions do I use?

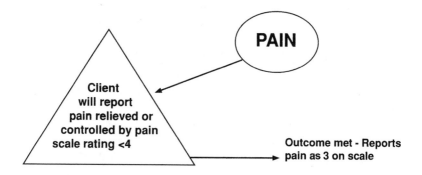

FIGURE 5.14   Was my outcome met?

individual maps, students have a better understanding of the complexity of client care than if no group interaction occurred. When students share their maps with other group members they often realize on their own where their deficits lie and are able as a group to come up with a more complete and accurate understanding of the intricacies of client care.

FLOW CHARTING

A similar concept, yet different from concept mapping, is flow charting. Flow charting requires students to look at an entire process by breaking it down into small sequential steps. As they examine each step, students are forced to question its need and value, thereby stimulating their intellectual processes. On completion of the flow chart, students not only understand the process more completely but have synthesized the knowledge of one process and are better able to apply it to another situation. A flow chart is a visual depiction of a procedure. It traces individual steps, provides a standard, and ensures a consistent plan for implementation. This visual conceptualization provides a reference for people who are unsure of the process, promotes quality by encouraging analysis that stimulates the continuous improvement process, and saves time by eliminating costly trial-and-error methods common in processes that are not well established.

Students in groups could be assigned a procedure to flow chart. In the clinical area, it may be a procedure that students have previously done, have observed staff nurses doing, or something that they will be required to do that particular clinical day. By completing the flow chart, students will better understand the process as well as the rationale for each step. It will serve as a better preparation method than merely reading the steps from a procedure book. Visualization of the process will stimulate their memory of key parts of the overall process. Figure 5.15 shows a completed flow chart depicting the process of drawing up a medication for intramuscular injection. By completing this process as a group, students become familiar with all the elements of preparing a medication for injection. They may find time-saving and safety-related strategies to improve this procedure that are not apparent to nurses completing this task on a routine basis. Students are required to think and use their intellectual and cognitive abilities to connect with the learning.

CONCEPT CASE ANALYSIS

Concept case analysis is a cognitive structure in which students are given a case situation and asked to pull from the case data, illustrating a specific concept. Students are also asked to develop interventions related to the data. Student groups are given a case as well as a chart outlining specific information to be retrieved from the case. They must fill in the data, first finding specifics in the case illustrating various parts of the concept, then determining appropriate interventions relevant to the client's needs. Tables 5.3 and 5.4 show an example using the concept of hazards of immobility in the case of a 32-year-old woman with rheumatoid arthritis. Students would first be challenged by the professor to discuss and complete the column "System/hazards" by listing common findings in this category. For example, under "Cardiovascular," common findings related to immobility are increased heart rate and orthostatic hypotension. Next, faculty should ask students to find data in the case on the hazards of immobility related to the cardiovascular system. Students would identify increased heart rate (120) and a low blood

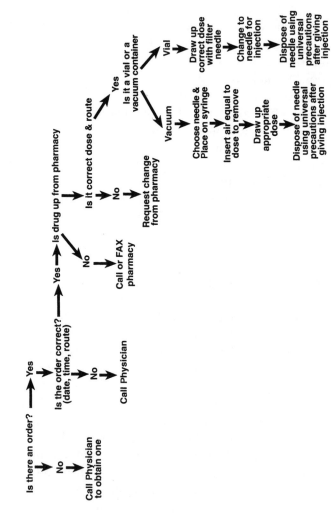

FIGURE 5.15 Flow chart example: Drawing up a medication for an IM injection.

TABLE 5.3   Concept Case Analysis

Case

Alice Williams is a 32-year-old white woman diagnosed with rheumatoid arthritis. She is 5 feet, 8 inches tall and weighs 110 pounds. She is a single mother with two preschoolers. She has been on bedrest for 3 weeks complaining of severe pain with any movement of her right ankle, left patella, and severe redness and swelling in the sacral area. Recently, she has been complaining of abdominal pain. Today's vital signs are T101, P120, R32, and BP 90/50.

Doctor's Orders

Naproxen, 375 mg tid
Plaquenil, 200 mg qd
Prednisone, 10 mg bid
Bactrim DS i hs
Iron Dextran 100 mg IM
Chair tid for 30 minutes

TABLE 5.4   Concept Case Analysis Chart

	Hazards of Immobility	
System/hazards	Data in the case	Nursing interventions
Musculoskeletal		
Integumentary		
Cardiovascular		
Respiratory		
Genitourinary		
Gastrointestinal		
Psychological		
Nutrition		

pressure (90/50) as significant findings for this category. In completing the intervention column, students should identify the potential risk of orthostatic hypotension and institute nursing measures of taking blood pressure in a lying and then sitting position, and then having the patient dangle her legs before getting out of bed. Students will be stimulated to find all the data and nursing implications related to this example.

Virtually any concept could be taken in its parts and used similarly in a case situation. For example, aspects of caring, components of self-concept, types of stress, functional patterns, and safety hazards are a few concepts that work well with cases. This strategy helps students structure their thinking and analytic skills and allows them to work together to enhance the depth of learning.

GAMES

There are multiple benefits for using games as a teaching strategy in both the classroom and clinical areas. Gaming structures meet all the necessary elements for learning nursing content. First, students are usually anxious about tests and this anxiety blocks their ability to process and retain information. Using games as a test review is fun, and reduces the anxiety and fear that often accompany test taking. Games also reduce the risk of failure, as grades are not given and learning occurs in a non-threatening environment. Second, games promote active student-centered learning, allowing students to interact freely as they solve problems. This strategy causes them to focus on concrete tasks and forces them to become engaged in learning the material. Active involvement enhances learning because students must give an answer and explain it, which stimulates their cognitive centers and helps lay down memory. Third, games provide immediate feedback, which gives students an open-ended opportunity to clarify their ideas, ask questions, and assess their own level of comprehension. Faculty can also evaluate student learning and clear up misconceptions. Fourth, games are highly motivating whereas teacher-delivered material is often tedious and boring. Fifth, games promote cooperation and social learning skills critical for team development. Each student has a part to perform and must stay alert and involved to play the game. Gaming encourages team spirit, which may stimulate students to study prior to the game so that they do not let their teammates down. Sixth, games are an excellent way to cover the content. Any information can be used to create a game. In general, games stimulate critical thinking, create community among the student groups, and cover the essential content.

When developing games faculty should determine what student outcomes they desire. Do they want students to learn just the facts, such as definitions, terminology, and lab values, or are they interested in involving students in higher-level cognitive thinking processes such as problem solving, prioritization, and application? It is likely that both of these aspects are desired (see Figure 5.16).

Games can be used in a variety of ways. They can be adapted to reinforce recall of information before in-depth discussion in class. This eliminates the need for educators to review facts in

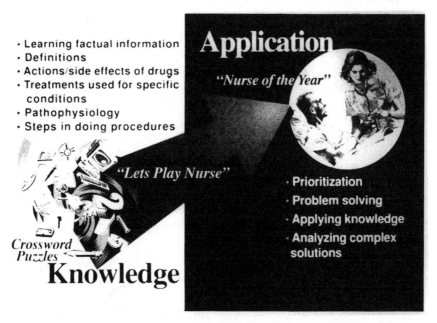

FIGURE 5.16 The versalitility of gaming—use for learning facts, applying knowledge, and everything in between.

lecture and reserves the time in class for processing of nursing content in relation to clinical situations. Games can be used as test review to help students prepare, process, recall, and remember information. Games can also be used by staff development educators as they conduct their yearly reviews regarding policy standards and basic competencies of the institution.

TIC-TAC TEST READY

As described by Glendon and Ulrich (1995), this game can be used with a small seminar of 15 students, or it can be adapted to larger classes. Each student's assignment before class is to review all reading and class notes on which they are to be tested and develop at least one test question per reading assignment or class period. Question format can vary as long as the response can be given verbally in a few words (true/false, fill in the blank, simple listing, multiple choice, etc.). The questions should reflect the most important content and be written on separate index cards and brought to class the day of the game. On game day, students are divided into five groups of three students each, providing there are only 15 students in the class. Before starting the game, each of the groups is required to take a portion of the questions, analyze them, delete any inappropriately stated questions, or modify them to read correctly. This is an important step in the process because students frequently lack skill in constructing test questions and by reviewing them as a group the students formulate the questions to become more succinct and pertinent. This activity also helps students analyze test questions and understand the reasoning behind the answers. Next, three of the five groups combine to form the nine squares of the tic-tac-toe board, which is drawn on the blackboard or overhead. Each of the nine students places his or her name in one of the squares. The remaining two groups (six students) compete in playing the traditional tic-tac-toe game. The professor serves as the game show host, score keeper, and judge. If the class is larger, students could be assigned these roles rather than the professor. Also, pairs of students rather than individual students could form the nine squares of the tic-tac-toe board, and the two groups playing the game could be larger than three students.

The game begins with a coin toss to determine which team goes first. The first team selects a square, and the person designated in that square asks the team one of the questions. The team has one minute to confer on the answer and respond. The student who researched the question validates the correctness of the answer. If this student misunderstands the material, the professor overrules the decision and explains the rationale for the correct answer. If the question is answered correctly, the team places an X in that square. If the team is incorrect, the opposing team is required to answer the same question correctly to place an O in the square. If neither team answers the question correctly, the square remains blank, and the judge explains the correct answer to the missed question. Teams take turns choosing squares, and the game continues until one team wins either three Xs or three Os in a straight or diagonal line. Rotation of team players and squares occurs at varying intervals, every two or three games, and continues until all the questions are exhausted or the class period ends.

As previously stated, this game can be played with many students by using teams to serve as the judge and teams to form the squares rather than individuals. Increasing the number of students on the teams who are the players is also a way to adapt the game to a larger group of students.

Because this is a game, prizes add to the competitive spirit and fun of the activity. The authors use candy to reward the winners; however, rewards also could include buttons; nursing professional supplies, such as pen lights and scissors; or even bonus points on tests. However, the use of bonus points is a controversial issue, and individual teachers need to determine the rewards appropriate for the activity.

LET'S PLAY NURSE

This game is based on the ideas and rules of "Bingo" and is used as a method for test review, although it could also be used as an overall NCLEX review. Students learn pertinent content and prepare for testing, yet enjoy themselves in the process.

As described by Ulrich and Glendon (1997), the first step in creating the game is to plan and write a variety of questions based on the same criteria used in planning any test. A good plan might be to model the test blueprint after the NCLEX format with questions on steps of the nursing process as well as questions related to safety, physiological integrity, psychosocial integrity, and health promotion. All questions need to have relatively short answers, yet incorporate analysis and application as well as recall (see Table 5.5). At least 100 questions writ ten on 3- × 5-inch cards with the questions on one side and the answers on the other are needed for a typical game. Faculty develop the questions for this game; however, students could create the questions as they study the content, which would compound the learning potential of the game. All of the question cards are placed in a large fishbowl in preparation for the student game.

TABLE 5.5   Questions for "Let's Play Nurse" Game

I.   *Analysis/Application*

1. A woman with placenta previa is admitted to Labor & Delivery. Assessment data show fetal heart rate of 100 and maternal BP of 80/40. What do you anticipate is happening?
   Answer: hemorrhage

2. Maria is 36-weeks pregnant, states her baby is not moving, and is scheduled for a non-stress test (NST). If the NST is nonreactive, what would you anticipate will happen next?
   Answer: contraction stress test (CST)

II.   *Recall*

1. Symptoms of pregnancy induced hypertension (PIH) include elevated blood pressure, edema, and _____.
   Answer: proteinuria

2. Symptoms are painless, bright red vaginal bleeding in the third trimester that increases in amount with each episode of bleeding.
   Answer: placenta previa

From Ulrich, D., & Glendon, K. (1997). Let's play nurse. *Nurse Educator, 22*(6), 9–10. Reprinted with permission.

The next step requires creating the nurse cards, much like Bingo cards (see Table 5.6). In creating the nurse cards, faculty randomly select question cards from the bowl and sequentially write one answer in each of the empty boxes on the nurse card. After returning the questions to the fishbowl, faculty repeat the same procedure to create each new nurse card. As many cards as needed for teams to play are developed. For example, in a class of 30 students, there could be six teams of five players each; therefore, the teacher would need six different nurse cards for the game.

Students are then divided into teams. Each team is given a nurse card. Questions are drawn from the fishbowl by the instructor or another student and posed to all teams. Teams are given 1 minute to discuss possible answers with their teammates. At that point, one team is called on to present answers to the question, generating a full class discussion. Only teams with the correct answer on their card are permitted to mark them. This process continues until one team yells "nurse," indicating a win with five

TABLE 5.6   Sample Nurse Card

N	U	R	S	E
		FREE		

correct answers in a row either on the diagonal, horizontal, vertical, or all four corners (see Table 5.7). In a final examination review, a coverall card could be required for a nurse win. The authors have developed this game in a variety of versions, highlighting nursing content in obstetrics, pediatrics, and fundamentals. For more information on the games, contact the authors (ulrichdl@ muohio.edu).

CROSSWORD PUZZLE COMPETITIONS

Crossword puzzles can be designed to cover information related to pathophysiology, knowledge of medications, or even nursing theorists. A strategy to make factual learning interesting and fun is to make completion of the puzzle a competition between student

TABLE 5.7   Sample of a Vertical Win Nurse Card

N	U	R	S	E
Muscle tone	Rhogam	Pregnancy Induced Hypertension (PIH)	Contraction Stress Test (CST)	Respirations
Elevated temperature	Abruptio placenta	Vaginal examinations	Pale or blue color	Apnea and bradycardia
Tachycardia	Neural tube defect	Free	Trendelenburg	Painless vaginal bleeding
Lecithin/ Sphingomyelin Ratio (L/S ratio)	Gavage	Painful vaginal bleeding	Broncho- pulmonary dysplasia (BPD)	Amniocentesis
Non-Stress Test (NST)	Placenta previa	Give calcium gluconate	Right occiput posterior (ROP)	Fetal lung maturity

groups. For example, instead of the teacher lecturing on the three Ps of diabetes—polyuria, polydipsia, and polyphagia—a crossword containing this information is used at the beginning of the class. Several minutes, as determined by the length of the puzzle, are allowed for student groups to finish their puzzle. It is optimal to either pair or use groups of three for this activity, as students need to be able to readily see the puzzle's across and down statements while sitting together and having only one puzzle. Once a student group is finished with the puzzle, those in the group raise their hands, or to add to the lively spirit of the game, groups could design their own signal to indicate completion of the task. To quickly verify correctness of the answer, the teacher uses an overhead transparency of a completed crossword and overlays the transparency on the student's answer sheet. If incorrect answers are detected, the game continues until another group accurately completes the puzzle. The first team that completes the puzzle correctly earns a prize as determined by the faculty.

Puzzle design is easily accomplished by creating statements for both the "across" and "down" sections of the puzzle and their answers. Computer programs are now available that automatically create the word blocks of the crossword, so most of the work lies in thinking about how to formulate the statements to fit a particular one-word answer. Examples of crosswords related to multiple topics are found in the current literature (Galuska, 1995; Lenaghan, 1996), or faculty members could devise their own (see Tables 5.8 and 5.9).

CROSSWORD COLLABORATIONS AND GRAND FINALE

Another variation on this same theme of using crosswords is to allow students to collaborate on the puzzles but eliminate the competitiveness of the game. Students collaborate in pairs or groups of three at the beginning of class on a crossword pertaining to previous reading assignments and the class content for the day. After a specified amount of time, the faculty member displays answers on an overhead transparency for students to check their

TABLE 5.8   Crossword Puzzle for Neurological Assessment

1	2	3 /	4	5	6	7	8	9	10	11	12	13	14	15	16
										R					
								V	A	L	S	A	L	V	A
D	E	C	A	D	R	O	N	N		C	P				
							A			C	I				
B	R	U	D	Z	I	N	S	K	I	O	N				
							O			O	A				
				A	S	P	I	R	I	N	L		F		
							H						A		
							A						C		C
			C	A	R	B	O	N	D	I	O	X	I	D	E
							Y						A		F
H	E	P	A	R	I	N							L		O
								G	L	A	S	C	O	W	T
							E								A
D	E	C	O	R	T	I	C	A	T	E					X
	E				H										I
	G				I										M
					R										E
					D										

results and make any corrections. Each week, a crossword is used to begin the class. By the end of the course, students have collected multiple crosswords containing essential facts that are of great use for test review. By using crosswords, faculty encourages students to be involved in learning important facts and processing this necessary information prior to class discussion. This activity enhances students' memory of the content and stimulates them to ask questions when class time begins. At the completion of the course, a portion of the final examination includes a comprehensive crossword puzzle containing a sample from each of the previously used crosswords. The use of this strategy helps students memorize important definitions and concepts that are needed before being required to apply the information to clinical nursing situations.

ULTIMATE MEMORY GAME

This game is based on the memory game of "Concentration." In the traditional game, the player turns over a playing piece and matches it to an identical piece. Initially, the player guesses the location of the match; then later, as pieces are turned over and shown, the player remembers the location of the piece that makes a match. This game follows the same premise, but an additional step is added. The student turns over a mnemonic and must match the corresponding definition of the mnemonic. When uncovering and matching mnemonics to their definition, students must verbally discuss their meaning (see Figure 5.17). After completing all matches, the players with the most matches win. This game could be played with several other different possibilities: medications (drug classes and their effects, drugs and their side effects, and drugs and their nursing implications); abbreviations and definitions; or names of diagnostic tests with nursing implications.

This is a quick game that reinforces memory of complex data. It can be used as a post-conference activity, as a study group aid, or as a class activity. The "drill" aspect of the activity enhances memory.

TABLE 5.9   Crossword Clues

Across

18	Intervention of exhale while turning patient prevents this
20	Medication that decreases cerebral swelling
25	Causes pain along the spine when flexed if abnormal
31	Oral drug commonly used in the prevention of strokes
43	Causes an increase in intracranial pressure
46	Intravenous drug used with stroke patients to prevent more clots from forming
49	Scale used to assess eye opening, motor, and verbal responses
57	Abnormal posture in which arms are flexed and legs are extended

Down

11	A sign of a basilar skull fracture, _____ eyes
19	Type of testing contraindicated if intracranial pressure high, _____ tap
21	Type of suctioning contraindicated if skull fracture present
33	Cranial nerve tested by asking patient to smile, frown, and puff out cheeks
41	Antibiotic given to treat meningitis
58	Withhold caffeine prior
59	Cranial nerve that tests pupillary response

INFO LINKS

Another game, "Info Links," is based on the classic "Dominoes" game. Each player or team is dealt six info cards. Each card is divided in half horizontally and contains a different word or meaning on each side (see Figure 5.18). The meanings and words on each card are unrelated. A few info cards may say "wild" on one side, and these can be used as any meaning or word the player wants it to represent. The remaining cards are put in a pile in the center of the table face down. To begin the game, the first player turns over the top card, and it begins as in the traditional Domino game. In turn, players try to add to the chain. If they do not have an information card that "fits," they must draw from the pile, increasing the number of cards they hold. If players can add to the chain, they must explain why that information card fits and get agreement from all group members. The first person or team

Abdominal Distention	<u>9 S's</u> Size Shape Surface Site Symptoms Softness Squeezability Spread Sensation	<u>8 F's</u> Fat Fluid Feces Flatus Fibroid Full bladder False pregnancy Fetus	Assessment of Cranial Nerve #3
Treatment of Sprain	Pain Assessment	Melanoma Characteristics	Assessment of Lump

<u>PQRST</u>
Problem Pain
Quality,
  Quantity
Region,
  Radiation
Signs,
  Symptoms
Time of
  Onset
	<u>RICE</u>
	Rest
	Ice
	Compress
	Elevate
		<u>PERRLA</u>
		Pupils
		Equal
		Round
		Reactive
		Light
		Accomodations
			<u>5 P's</u>
			Pallor
			Pain
			Paresthesia
			Pulses
			Poikeothermy

<u>ABCD</u>
Asymmetry
  of Border
Bleeding
Color—blue
  black
  variegated
Diameter↑6
  cm
	Wound
	assessement
		Circulation
		checks
			<u>REEDA</u>
			Redness
			Edema
			Ecchymosis
			Discharge
			Approximation

FIGURE 5.17   Examples of cards for the ultimate memory game.

Info Links

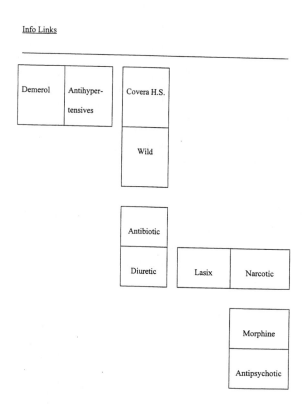

FIGURE 5.18   Info links.

out of information cards wins. This game of Info Links is an excellent way to drill students on specific medications and their classifications, laboratory tests and nursing implications, or medical terminology and their definitions, to name a few.

NAME IT

This is a game that is based on the old television show, "Name That Tune." In preparation for the game, the professor or groups of students pick a concept, a historical nurse leader, a theorist, a complication, or other such entity. They create a list of clues that describe their concept or person, listing them from general to

TABLE 5.10   Example of "Name It" Clues

Placenta Previa

1. Vaginal bleeding is a symptom.
2. A complication of pregnancy.
3. It occurs during the third trimester.
4. It may require a cesarean section.
5. The bleeding is painless and bright red.
6. It can be partial, complete, or low lying.

Florence Nightingale

1. A historical nurse leader.
2. Believed nursing education should occur in a university setting.
3. Responsible for the first attempts at nursing research.
4. Nursed soldiers in the Crimean War.
5. Stressed cleanliness and environmental conditions in nursing.
6. Lady with the lamp.

specific. A list of 6 to 10 clues per entity works well. Once a number of these has been created, student groups play the game (see Table 5.10 for an example). The "host" of the game, who could be the teacher or a student, and two student groups play the game. A coin toss determines which group begins. A designated speaker from each group comes forward. The speaker from the group going first says, "My group can 'name it' in five clues." The other group's speaker can then say, "My group can 'name it' in four clues." This back-and-forth challenge continues until one group's speaker declines the challenge and says, "name it." The host then gives the other team the appropriate number of clues. They have 60 seconds to discuss the answer among themselves before the host asks the group's speaker to "name it." If they answer correctly, they get a point. If they answer incorrectly, the other team gets a chance to answer. If they answer correctly, they get the point. If they also miss, the host reads the remaining clues, and the first team to respond correctly gets the point. After each point is scored, a class discussion evolves about the entity being described. The team with the most points wins.

This is an excellent way for students to prepare for an examination or practice their skills of memory and identification.

WHAT'S THAT INTERVENTION?

This game is based on the television show, "Family Feud." Teams of four to six students play the game, two teams at a time. A student or the professor serves as the host and asks the questions. Any student can serve as the one who reveals the answers as they are discovered. Before the game, the professor or student groups develop several nursing situations that require numerous interventions (see Table 5.11), and using an overhead transparency record the interventions and then cover the list so it is not visible to the players. Teams form a row on opposite sides of the host. One at a time, members come forward to represent their team. The host reads the scenario, and the first member who rings the bell sitting on the table in front of the host is eligible to respond with one intervention. If he or she is correct, this person may either choose to have the team complete the intervention list or pass it to the other team to solve. If wrong, the other team gets a chance. The host then asks each member of the team that is answering, in turn, to give an appropriate intervention. If it is on the list, it is

TABLE 5.11   Examples of "What's That Intervention?" Situation

Situation: Jill Southern is 2 days postop from an abdominal hysterectomy. She is complaining of chills, is perspiring profusely, and says she feels "awful." In checking her dressing you note redness, edema, and small amounts of yellow purulent discharge. What do you do?

1. Take vitals—especially temperature
2. Call doctor
3. Change clothes
4. Keep culture of drainage for lab
5. Change dressing
6. Offer fluids
7. Document findings
8. Check laboratory values (i.e., white blood cell count)

uncovered, and the next member gets a turn. If the team gets three "strikes" or incorrect responses before uncovering all of the answers, the other team gets to collaborate and decide jointly on one intervention thought to be on the list. If this team chooses one on the list, these group members can steal the total points for that scenario. Teams accumulate points based on the number of interventions they uncover. After three scenarios, the team with the most points wins. After each scenario, the instructor leads a class discussion on what interventions are appropriate, their rationale, and potential complications.

This game is also an excellent preparation for course examinations, NCLEX, or just review. It could be used by staff development or nursing supervisors as review for staff or preparation for certification examinations or hospital accreditation.

MEDICATION MADNESS

This game can be played by two groups of students in a classroom situation or by pairs of students in a clinical group. The faculty member puts the names of numerous medications on 3- × 5-inch cards and places them in a small paper or cloth bag. Posted on the board or on an overhead, the instructor lists the things students need to remember about medications, such as classification, normal dosage and route, physiological action, side effects, and nursing implications. One team or pair draws a card. They read the name of the medication and give an answer to one of the categories listed on the overhead or board. If they cannot come up with an answer, the other team or pair gets the chance to respond. The faculty member writes his or her answer next to the appropriate item on the list and asks the rest of the class to respond to its correctness. If it is correct, the other team or pair gives the answer to another item on the list. Discussion follows. This continues until all items asked for on the board or overhead are filled in. At this point, the medication is reviewed by the class. A new card is drawn, and the process is repeated. Each team or pair gets one point for every correct reply. The winner is the team or pair with the highest number of points.

This activity is an excellent way to review pertinent medications related to content area in the classroom or clinical unit. It stimulates discussion related to nursing implications and allows students to create and visually view important aspects necessary to know about specific medications. This enhances memory as students are active in the process of learning.

NURSE OF THE YEAR

"Nurse of the Year" is a great game to play with a few students. It is a good post-conference activity and can be designed in a variety of ways to elicit the content learning and thinking skills desired. In a small group, students play the game as the instructor serves as moderator and judge. The object of the game is to move a player piece from "Novice Nurse" to "Nurse of the Year." Players, in turn, roll a die and move the corresponding number of spaces on the game board. As players land on a space they must draw the designated card and answer the question correctly in order to remain on that space. An incorrect answer requires them to return to their prior location on the board. A few spaces do not require the student to answer a question. The instructor leads the discussion of each question, adds pertinent information students neglect to mention, and clarifies or corrects incorrect responses. One game board can be used with different card sets to tailor the learning to the objectives set by the teacher (see Figure 5.19). Table 5.12 shows examples of cards that might be used in game. In this example, the "S cards" reflect situations that might occur in the life of a registered nurse and direct the player to move ahead or back on the game board, or to miss a turn. "LE cards" reflect legal-ethical dilemmas a nurse might experience, "C cards" situations that require communication skills, and "P cards" physiological concerns. Additional cards could be added to reflect management/ leadership skills, nursing interventions, or other areas pertinent to student learning needs. The game could be played with more students by having pairs of students compete with other pairs. It can be adapted to serve the teaching needs of the faculty member and the learning needs of the student.

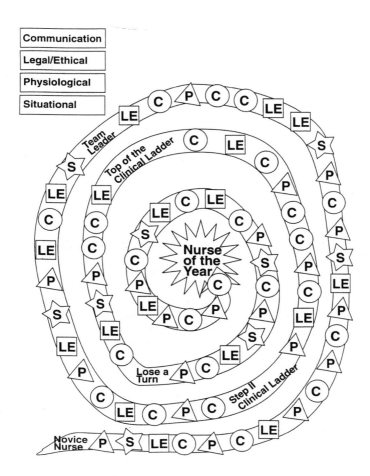

FIGURE 5.19   **Nurse of the Year game board.**

THINK LIKE A NURSE

"Think Like a Nurse" is a game developed to encourage critical thinking and help students learn essential content in nursing subject areas. The game, played in groups, is a vehicle to help students process solutions to problems they may encounter in clinical practice. The game board consists of a path from the start to the end of the game (Figure 5.20). The path is composed of four different

TABLE 5.12   Examples of Cards for "Nurse of the Year" Game

LE Cards	Your 50-year-old client has been diagnosed with terminal cancer. The doctor tells you that the family does not want her to know the diagnosis. She is coherent and begins asking you questions about the diagnosis. What do you do?
	You witness a peer stealing codeine from the medicine cart. She tells you that she has migraines and cannot work without codeine. Her doctor refuses to give her enough codeine to allow her to work comfortably. She begs you not to turn her in and promises never to do it again. What do you do?
S Cards	• You were late to work; go back three spaces. • You forgot to update your cardiopulmonary resuscitation and liability insurance; go back five spaces. • You just presented a great staff development program; go to "Step 2 Clinical Ladder." • You got a merit raise; move forward two spaces.
P cards	A 56-year-old white man is postop for a carotid angiogram. His R femoral dressing is dry and intact and without swelling. R pedal pulse is strong and regular. As he is consuming his clear liquid diet, he dribbles the fluid out of his mouth, and you observe facial weakness. Anticipate what could be happening and other data you need to collect.
C Cards	You arrive at work and find you are the only RN for 30 postop clients. An LPN and aide are your only staff. Both are new employees and tell you they can handle only two patients each. Your supervisor tells you to "Get used to it—that's life!"
	It is 3 a.m., and your 10-hour postop nephrectomy client has a pulse of 120, blood pressure of 80/60, and a hemoglobin of 6. He is restless and complaining of severe back pain. You call the doctor, and she instructs you to "keep an eye on him and report back to me in the morning." How do you respond? What do you do?

colored squares. For publication purposes the illustration shows the colors in shades of gray rather than four primary colors. The object is to move from the start to the end of the game by answering questions from different categories based on the color of the squares. For example, in the medical-surgical version the four

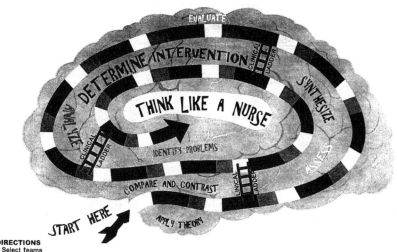

DIRECTIONS
• Select teams
• Roll dice
• Move to space
• Answer question according to shape or space
• If correct remain on space
• If incorrect, go back to previous space
• Use clinical ladder if available & advance ahead
• First team to finish Thinks Like a Nurse

FIGURE 5.20   "Think Like a Nurse."

areas would be medical nursing, surgical nursing, medications, and potpourri (Table 5.13). The students can play in small clinical groups or the entire classroom could be divided into sub-groups prior to playing the game. To determine which sub-group begins the game, a representative of each rolls a die once. The sub-group with the highest number goes first, followed by the one with the next highest number, and so forth in sequence. To begin the game one member of one sub-group rolls a die for his or her sub-group and moves the number of spaces indicated on the die. The faculty member asks a question from that category. The sub-group has two minutes to collectively arrive at a solution or answer to the question. At the same time, the remaining sub-groups also discuss the question and determine their solutions. After the allotted two minutes of discussion time, the faculty member asks the members of the sub-group that threw the die to reveal their answer to the entire class. An overall discussion ensues with all sub-groups detail-

TABLE 5.13   Sample Questions for Medical-Surgical Think Like a Nurse Game

Medical Nursing

1. A client in chronic renal failure should limit what in his or her diet and why?
2. Your diabetic client has a blood glucose of 300 mg/dl. What would be your recommendations regarding exercise at this time and why?

Surgical Nursing

1. What is the purpose of an NG tube after a cholecystectomy?
2. What nursing interventions are appropriate in caring for a client postoperatively to prevent the complication of thrombophlebitis?

Medications

1. What is the antibiotic of choice against tetanus?
2. What teaching is indicated for a client put on prazosin (minipress) 1 mg. po daily?

Potpourri

1. What four elements must a client prove in order to claim malpractice?
2. Your client has had frequent urinary tract infections. She asks if there is anything she can do to prevent these or at least decrease their frequency. What would you tell her?

ing their varied solutions. When all solutions have been presented and discussed, the entire class determines whether the initial sub-group answered the question sufficiently to remain on its occupied square. A simple show of hands will suffice. The game continues as each sub-group rolls the die, moves the appropriate spaces, and answers the question adequately. The game may continue until a sub-group reaches the end of the path first and wins or until the time allotted for the game is exhausted. In the latter case the sub-group that has progressed farthest on the game board is declared the winner. This game is an excellent way to involve students in discussing common clinical situations that affect professional nurses as they fulfill the complex role of caring for clients. An added bonus to the game is the community it creates among students as they collectively play the game. The aspect of relationship building by having fun together is lacking among most student groups but is essential in assisting them to learn to work collaboratively. The authors have developed several versions of this game (obstetrics, medical-surgical, and nurse educator) and can be contacted for more information.

MUSICAL N-U-R-S-E

Students stand in a circular fashion and music is played as a ball is passed from one student to the next. When the music stops the student who is holding the ball asks a question from a stack of questions in the center of the circle. The first student who steps forward into the middle of the circle has the opportunity to answer the question. If the student answers the question correctly, he or she is awarded a card with an N on it. If the student answers incorrectly, he or she does not receive the N card and another student has the chance to earn the letter by shouting out the answer. The game continues until one student has earned all five letter cards to spell the word NURSE. Questions can be provided by the faculty member or students can be asked to bring questions to class the day the game is to be played. When students formulate questions to ask to their peers, they must articulate the rationale for the answer, a process that increases retention and understanding far more than passively receiving this information through a lecture. It is the faculty's responsibility to assure that all students clearly understand the rationale for the correct answer. Virtually any content can be covered in an enjoyable and interactive way.

ISOLATION CHALLENGE

This game is ideal for covering content related to infection control such as isolation technique, universal precautions, types of isolation, blood-borne pathogens, and infectious diseases. Students are divided into teams. As a team they pick one member to be the team mascot. This student dresses in isolation garb: gown, mask, head and shoe covering, and gloves. At this point the faculty member asks each team a question sequentially. The team has two minutes to interact and answer the question. Total class discussion follows each question. If the team cannot answer the question correctly, its mascot must remove one item of isolation garb. At this point faculty must intervene to ensure that students understand the correct response. When the mascot has no isolation garb remaining, the team is eliminated from the competition. The team who has the most isolation garb items remaining wins.

This chapter has presented numerous ways to involve students experientially by tapping them holistically through their vision, hearing, emotions, and intellect. All of the strategies presented enhance critical thinking abilities and encourage the retention of content. Their ease of use allows the faculty flexibility as they plan their classes to include interactive group learning.

CHAPTER 6

Writing as a Tool for Critical Thinking

Effective communication involves more than being able to express oneself verbally. Students need to be articulate in writing as well as in speaking. Writing allows students to formulate their own ideas and create a logical flow of thoughts. It also teaches them how to use words appropriately, build their vocabulary, and practice effective writing skills. When students are required to put their thoughts in writing, it forces them to reflect on their own ideas. It makes them consider their own value structures as well as analyze and critique the logic of their thinking processes. As nursing faculty, we must help students practice and perfect this essential communication skill. As we develop activities that challenge students to use their skills in writing, it is important to remember that students will do better if they have a structured format and can see examples of well-written journals or papers (Ibarreta & McLeod, 2004). This chapter describes several techniques useful for implementing this learning outcome.

GROUP WRITING STRUCTURE: PASS THE WRITING

Traditional scholarly papers graded by faculty are but one way to help students perfect their writing skills. Group writing intensifies the learning as peers read and critique each other's writing. It provides the writer with suggestions to improve clarity, logic, and flow of ideas and gives additional supportive viewpoints or rebuttal. Oftentimes students feel less threatened by peer critique and more supported as they work together to improve their individual skills. Faculty can transform traditional individual writing exercises into a group structure by first giving individual group members a topic or prompt to write about as a homework assignment or class activity. Each group could be given different topics to explore. On completion of the individual writing exercise, each group member passes his or her writing to another peer who belongs to a different group and has responded to a different topic or prompt. The peer who receives the writing must respond with a written critique. Asking students to critique requires that the instructor first help them learn how to do this skill effectively. Providing them with a written guide to record their perceptions helps demystify this new student role. The critique should include a variety of common categories based on actual writing skills and the writer's ideas and values (see Table 6.1). The writing and critique are then returned to the original writer, who shares it with his or her group members (who have all written on the same topic). Group members combine, synthesize, and summarize their individual ideas on their assigned topic into one group paper through consensus. Each group then summarizes its main points in an overall class presentation and discussion. Both group and individual papers are then collected by the faculty member for grading or constructive criticism. This group writing format, Pass the Writing, provides a framework for faculty to use to implement group writing in their classes. It can be used in its totality, as described earlier, or adapted to the situation (see Table 6.2).

WRITING PROMPTS

The following are examples of topics or writing prompts that stimulate critical analysis related to nursing practice.

Clinical Writing Prompts

Table 6.3 gives several examples of writing prompts that could be used as an ending to a clinical experience. Because most clinical

TABLE 6.1   Peer Critique of Written Assignments

	NA	1	2	3	4
1. The values expressed are congruent with nurse practice act.					
2. Correct and logical interpretations exist throughout the paper.					
3. Sentence structure (complete sentences, no run-ons) is correct.					
4. Topic sentence exists for each paragraph.					
5. Correct grammar is used.					
6. Correct punctuation is used.					
7. There is a logical flow of ideas/reasoning/assumptions.					
8. The paper has clarity—it is clear and makes sense.					
9. The summary clearly pulls together the total paper.					
10. The body of the paper supports the topic sentence.					
11. The writer adequately completed the writing prompt.					

Comments—strengths and suggestions for improving the paper:

Critiquer's personal response to the essence of the paper:

Writer _____
Critiquer _____

Key: NA = not applicable; 1 = rarely; 2 = sometimes; 3 = usually; 4 = always.

groups consist of only 8 to 10 students and conferences are relatively short, the same writing prompt may be used for everyone. Students could pass their written work to the right or left, as they sit in a circle, for critiquing. These assignments could be given during pre-conference activity so students could reflect on them

TABLE 6.2   Group Writing Structure: Pass the Writing

1. Each group is given a different topic or prompt to write about.
2. Each group member individually completes the writing assignment.
3. Each member passes his or her individual writing to a peer in another group for critique.
4. Peers respond with a written critique based on specific criteria (see Table 6.1).
5. The critique is returned to the original writer.
6. Original group members meet and share their individual writing and its critique.
7. Members of each group combine everyone's ideas into a "group" writing on the assigned topic.
8. Groups report to the entire class and summarize main points.
9. Faculty grades or critiques the final writing products.

TABLE 6.3   Using Clinical-Writing Prompts

Writing Prompts

Write about your own development as a nurse after today's clinical experience

1. Give five examples of your growth as a person and a professional.
2. What's the best thing that happened today, and why?
3. What's the worst thing that happened today, and how did you respond to it?
4. Give two new points you learned today that you will use in your future practice.
5. List two positive things the staff nurse you worked with did that you intend to emulate.
6. List two negative things the staff nurse you worked with did that you are certain you will never do.

throughout the clinical experience or given as a post-conference activity. Instead of completing the entire process as explained in Table 6.2, the exercise could be adapted to save time by assigning pairs of students to correspond and critique each other's work via e-mail. Students learn how to record their ideas effectively, as well as how to critique others' writing abilities, ultimately learning or improving their own writing skills.

Writing Prompts to Increase Insight and Perspective

An example of a way to challenge students who often have narrowly confined paradigms or lack of diversity in their ideas is for faculty to require students to react to many different situations through writing (see Table 6.4). Through this type of writing exercise, students will begin to learn how their personal values and feelings related to differences might affect their nursing care or their working relationships. As student groups use the Pass the Writing structure (see Table 6.2), they will, it is hoped, develop insight into their own personal prejudices and broaden their thinking so that they can view the world from a variety of perspectives. This exercise could be used for small groups both in the classroom and in clinical areas, and could be combined with another strategy, Academic Controversy (see Chapter 3), to add yet another dimension to the learning. Being exposed to opposing viewpoints and arguments helps students learn to appreciate perspectives different from their own.

TABLE 6.4   Using Writing Prompts to Increase Insight and Perspectives Related to Different Paradigms

Write your reaction to

1. Nurses who make errors in medications and procedures.
2. Male nurses who work in obstetrics.
3. Chemically dependent nurses who still practice.
4. People who live on welfare.
5. Parents who abuse their children.
6. Women who place their children for adoption.
7. Women who abuse drugs while pregnant.
8. Mentally ill practicing nurses.
9. Women who have abortions.
10. People with human immunodeficiency virus.
11. Homosexual patients or nurses.
12. Patients who are racist.
13. Nurses who fail state boards.

Writing Prompts to React to Reading Assignments

Often faculty ask students to read recent journal articles, research articles, or newspaper editorials. Traditionally, faculty have used the annotated bibliography format to assure that students have read material assigned. However, is it that we want to be sure the reading is read, or are we really wanting the student to understand, critique, and reflect on the author's work? The use of one or more writing prompts that focus on the critical thinking skills of analysis or developing insight into the author's assumptions can increase students' depth of learning and make the article more meaningful (see Table 6.5). These prompts require critical thinking rather than allow students merely to copy abstracts or findings.

Students learn to read critically and then express their analysis in written form as well as how to respond to another's analysis in an organized, thoughtful way. By using the Pass the Writing structure, students learn not only to think critically and critique, but also gain important knowledge from the information in the articles themselves. Stretching students' thinking and requiring them actually to analyze and critique the author's assumptions results in a higher level of discussion when readings are covered in class, or when students are asked to complete a group problem-solving activity based on the readings.

TABLE 6.5   Writing Prompts to Stimulate Critical Thinking in Relation to Assigned Articles/Readings

1. Summarize the reading in three sentences.
2. What are two major assumptions of the author?
3. After reading the article, what questions would you like to ask the author?
4. How could you use this information in your future nursing practice?
5. Did you agree with author or not, and why?
6. What additional ideas do you have that would support the author's viewpoint?
7. Write a rebuttal to the article/reading.
8. Explain the essence of the article to your classmate or a nursing colleague.

USING GRAPHS AND INFORMATION
AS THINKING PROMPTS

Students need to learn to interpret data from charts, graphs, and other visually displayed information as well as how to use written factual information to create these visual interpretations. Developing these skills is a part of learning to express data in a written form. One way to help students develop these skills is to give them examples of charts or graphs that present factual data and ask them in groups to write a narrative description interpreting the chart or graph examples. They could also be given a narrative explanation of facts and asked to do the opposite: display the data visually in charts or graphs. Using the same template as in Pass the Writing, students could pass the graph/information. The skill of being able to explain charts or graphs and the ability to develop them are important to ensuring total understanding of the information. Also, being able to dialogue with others who have either interpreted the data differently or chosen to display it in a different manner helps students realize the importance of accurately explaining or depicting data. Table 6.6 and Figures 6.1 and 6.2 give fictional examples of both processes; however, actual data could be obtained from sources such as research articles or student surveys, if the instructor wishes. A variation of this activity could involve students in constructing, administering, and collating data, and depicting their results with both narrative and visual illustrations. This class project would give them practice in learning to write appropriate and clear questions as well as explain their results to others in clear, concise terms and visual depictions.

CASES AS WRITING PROMPTS FOR APPLICATION

Application is a skill faculty hopes that students will develop as a result of listening to lectures, reading textbook assignments and research articles, and practicing clinically. Sometimes this connection is not readily apparent to some students, who tend to view clinical situations and classroom experiences as separate entities.

TABLE 6.6   Examples of Narrative Information for Students to Chart or Graph

1. Healthy Home Care saw 873 clients last year. The ages of the clients range from 3 months to 96 years old. Twenty-four were 6 months of age or younger, 16 were 6 months to 18 months old, 8 were 2 years old, 47 were 53 years old, 62 were 81 years old, 76 were 64 years old, 121 were 73 years old, 61 were 60 years old, 96 were 77 years old, and 116 were 68 years old. Illustrate these data visually.
2. The following are the raw data from a survey done on 100 patients on a surgical unit related to pain relief. Illustrate these results.

	Always	Often	Sometimes	Rarely	Never
My nurse asked me to rate my pain on a scale of 0 to 10.	10	20	40	15	15
My nurse medicated me when my pain exceeded 5 on a scale of 0 to 10.	44	33	25	0	0
My nurse asked me if the medication worked after administering it.	31	14	20	25	10
My nurse prepared and administered my pain medications in a timely manner.	7	5	10	10	68

Faculty can use writing to strengthen this connection and reinforce students' ability to apply theory and research to clinical practice. Table 6.7 gives an example of a case study in which students are asked to apply concepts related to theory. This could be implemented in the classroom using the group-writing structure, Pass the Writing. Faculty could develop case studies to illustrate a variety of concepts, such as chronic illness, family, developmental processes, teaching and learning, caring, or just one specific concept related to a nursing theorist (i.e., self-care, adaptation, conservation, etc.). Being able first to understand a concept and then actually use it in a case situation extends the student's learning

- Write a narrative explanation of this graph
- What other information do you need?
- What are your conclusions?

FIGURE 6.1   **Examples of graphs using fictional data for students to explain.**

and depth of comprehension. Application exercises etch concepts into the student's mind and enhance memory and future abilities to use the information. Again, writing prompts serve to expand the learning process by requiring students to think critically and relate concepts to real-life situations.

PRACTICE PROBLEMS AS WRITING PROMPTS

As nurses, students will be required to solve many complex problems involving clients or staff. The first step in solving a particular problem is to determine the cause. Table 6.8 lists several examples of problems students may encounter as practicing professional nurses. Faculty can use these problems as the basis for students to analyze individually and determine causes and plausible solutions in writing. After individually recording their thoughts, students

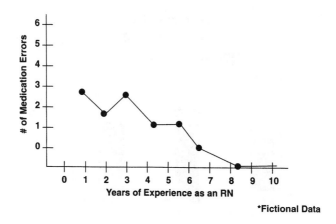

• **Explain in writing your conclusions related to this graph.**
• **What other data do you need?**

FIGURE 6.2 Examples of graphs using fictional data for students to explain.

TABLE 6.7   Case Study for Students to Apply a Principle/Theory To

Joe Sweet is a 78-year-old insulin-dependent diabetic. He lives alone with his dog, Barky—his only companion. His son, Sam, who lives nearby does not know what to do with him, as he eats only once a day and frequently has periods of hypoglycemia. Last week, Sam found Joe lying at the bottom of the stairs. His only injury appears to be a gash on his toe, where his toenail was ripped off. Sam has contacted a nursing home, but Joe refuses to leave his home because of Barky.

Complete one of the following:

1. Apply a nursing theorist of your choice to this situation.
2. Apply developmental theory to this situation.
3. Apply family theory to this situation.
4. Apply chronic illness theory to this situation.
5. Apply pathophysiology of diabetes to this situation.

TABLE 6.8   Common Problems Encountered by Practicing Professional Nurses

1. Staff nurses are refusing to care for clients getting abortions on an obstetrical unit in a major university hospital.
2. An AIDS patient is being ignored by the nursing staff as evidenced by the patient's report.
3. Staff nurses are restraining all confused elderly clients despite existing restraint policies.
4. A nurse observes her peer charting administration of gentamycin at a time other than when she did it, which will affect the drug blood level.
5. Staff nurses think an inadequate RN/patient ratio exists for safe care on their unit.
6. Dr. Doe demands that povidone-iodine be used to cleanse and heal a wound when recent research recommends a hydrocolloid dressing.

can critique and respond to each other's responses, combine and expand their ideas, discuss alternative causes and solutions, or, as a group, come to a consensus on the feasibility of the success of the chosen solution. Again, the group-writing structure, Pass the Writing, provides a framework for student groups to process and expand their ideas. Allowing students to first think about, then write about, and then discuss with others the common problems and frustrations faced by nursing professionals will give them practice in group problem solving.

BENEFITS

There are many benefits to using writing as an individual exercise, but group writing intensifies and multiplies the benefits. In the group-writing process, individual students must first formulate their own ideas and record them in a way so that others will understand their meaning. They must then critique the work of others, another aspect of thinking critically. Students who critique learn how to use specific criteria to evaluate written work and formulate their own evaluative ideas in written form. As a group, students formulate a final product that contains ideas from all members and expands the overall depth of thinking and number of thoughts that result in a better overall writing sample. Students learn to think about their own thinking (Paul, 1993; Paul & Elder, 2001) in relation to their own writing as well as the writing of others. They learn to summarize or explain information, organize their thoughts logically, and explain and illustrate data. The use of writing has many possibilities in all aspects of critical thinking and is vital to the overall development of the professional nurse. The group-writing structure, Pass the Writing provides a basis for writing activities. It is meant to serve as a template; however, faculty can adapt it to fit individual class time and learning objectives.

Epilogue

The idea of interactive group learning is becoming more and more popular in higher education as well as in the field of nursing. There is an abundance of literature praising the attributes of active learning, yet few sources provide the faculty member with instructions on how to implement it in nursing classrooms and clinical conferences. This book has conceptualized the idea of interactive group learning by explaining a variety of strategies the nurse educator can use in the classroom and clinical areas. As experienced educators we have learned that merely embracing the idea of interaction does not necessarily guarantee success in its implementation. We have two final tips that will ease your transition to group learning and ultimately enhance the learning potential of your students, as well as stimulate you to broaden your repertoire of teaching techniques. First, remember that **balance is the key**. You don't have to completely abandon your lecture methods. Creating a balance among group methods, lecturing, and other creative experiential strategies will keep your students interested and increase their learning potential. Use several different techniques to vary the atmosphere of your classroom presentations. Students' attention spans require a change of pace at least every twenty minutes. Remember that the more senses you involve in the activity, the greater the retention. Second, **don't just let things happen**. Planning is paramount whether you are preparing for a class or clinical post-conference. Just because students will be "discovering" their own knowledge does not mean the role of the expert is not needed. Use the comprehensive group learning model as a blueprint for your learning design. this model will ensure that you have considered the importance of critical thinking, cooperative learning, and experiential learning in planning learning activities. As you gain confidence in your abilities to teach in this new modality and expand your knowledge of teaching and learning strategies, our hope is that you will create your own interactive strategies and share them with other nurse educators through presentations and publications.

References

Alfaro-LeFevre, R. (1994). Teaching nurses critical thinking. *Academy of Medical-Surgical Nurses News*, 4–8.

Angelo, T. A., & Cross, K. P. (1993). *Classroom assessment techniques: A handbook for college teachers* (2nd ed.). San Francisco: Josey-Bass.

Aronson, E., Blaney, C., Stephen, C., Sikes, J., & Snapp, M. (1978). *The jigsaw classroom*. Beverly Hills, CA: Sage.

Aumiller, L., & Rudloff, G. (1986). Decentralization reduces absenteeism. *Journal of Nursing Administration, 16*, 16–30.

Bandman, E. L., & Bandman, B. (1995). *Critical thinking in nursing*. Norwalk, CT: Appleton & Lange.

Barr, R., & Tagg, J. (1995). From teaching to learning: A new paradigm for undergraduate education. *Change, 27*, 13–25.

Beitz, J. (1997). Concept mapping. Paper presented at the Nursing Education '97 Conference, Allegheny University, Philadelphia, PA.

Beitz, J. (1998). Concept mapping-navigating the learning process. *Nurse Educator, 23*(5), 35–41.

Bevis, E. (1989). Clusters of influence for practical decision making about curriculum. In E. Bevis & J. Watson (Eds.), *Toward a caring curriculum: A new pedagogy for nursing* (pp. 107–152). New York: National League for Nursing.

Bigge, M. L. (1971). *Learning theories for teachers* (2nd ed.). New York: Harper & Row.

Bonwell, C., & Eison, J. (1991). Active learning: Creating excitement in the classroom (ASHE-ERIC Higher Education Report No. 1). Washington, DC: The George Washington University School of Education & Human Development.

Brookfield, S. (1989). *Developing critical thinkers: Challenging adults to explore alternative ways of thinking and acting*. San Francisco: Jossey-Bass.

Browne, M., & Keeley, S. (1990). *Asking the right questions*. Upper Saddle River, NJ: Prentice Hall.

Centre Productions. (1984). *Special care* (videorecording). Madison, WI: Wisconsin Educational Communications Board.

Cohen, E. (1994). *Status treatment for the classroom* (videotape manual). New York: Teachers College Press.

Cooper, J. L., & Mueck, R. (1990). Student involvement in learning: Cooperative learning and college instruction. *Journal on Excellence in College Teaching, 1*, 68–76.

Cooper, J., Prescott, S., Cook, L., Smith, L., Mueck, R., & Cuseo, J. (1990). *Cooperative learning and college instruction: Effective use of student learning teams.* Carson: California State University.

Cross, K., & Angelo, T. (1988). *Classroom assessment techniques: A handbook for faculty.* Ann Arbor, MI: National Center for Research to Improve Post Secondary Teaching and Learning.

Cross, K. P., & Steadman, M. H. (1996). *Classroom research: Implementing the scholarship of teaching.* San Francisco: Jossey-Bass.

Cuseo, J. (1992). Cooperative learning versus small group discussions and group projects: The critical differences. *Cooperative Learning in College Teaching, 2,* 5–6, 8.

Dailey, M. (1992). Developing case studies. *Nurse Educator, 17,* 8–10.

Dale, E. (1969). *Audiovisual methods in teaching* (3rd ed.). New York: Holt, Rinehart, & Winston.

Daley, B. (1996). Concept maps: Linking nursing theory to clinical nursing practice. *Journal of Continuing Education in Nursing, 27,* 17–27.

Daley, B. J. (1999). Concept maps: A strategy to teach and evaluate critical thinking. *Journal of Nursing Education, 38*(1), 42.

Dewey, J. (1944). *Democracy and education: An introduction to the philosophy of education.* New York: Macmillan.

DiFeliciantonio, T. (Producer and director). (1986). *Living with AIDS* (video-recording). Urbana, IL: Carle Medical Communications.

Ekwall, E. (1976). *Diagnosis and remediation of the disabled reader.* Boston: Allyn & Bacon.

Ennis, R. H. (1989). Critical thinking and subject specificity: Clarification and needed research. *Educational Research, 18*(3), 4–10.

Facione, N. C., Facione, P. A., & Sanchez, C. A. (1994). Critical thinking disposition as a measure of competent clinical judgement: The development of the California Critical Thinking Disposition Inventory. *Journal of Nursing Education, 33*(8), 345–350.

Feingold, C., Calaluce, M., & Kallen, M. (2004). Computerized patient model and simulated clinical experiences: Evaluation with baccalaureate nursing students. *Journal of Nursing Education, 43*(4), 156–162.

Frederick, P. (1990). The power of the story and emotions in motivating students. Paper presented at the 10th Annual Lilly Conference on College Teaching, Oxford, OH.

Frierson, H. (1986). Two intervention methods: Effects on groups of predominantly Black nursing students' board scores. *Journal of Research & Development in Education, 19,* 18–23.

Galuska, L. (1995). Solve the puzzle of pediatric cardiopulmonary failure. *MCN, 20,* 334–336, 340.

Gandolfi, E., Tringali, S., & Cole, R. (producers), & Tringali, S. (director). (1985). *Don't cry for me* (videorecording). Brookline, MA: Umbrella Films.

Glendon, K., & Ulrich, D. (1992a). Using cooperative learning strategies. *Nurse Educator, 17,* 37–40.

Glendon, K., & Ulrich, D. (1992b). Using cooperative decision making strategies in nursing practice. *Nursing Administration Quarterly, 17,* 69–73.

Glendon, K., & Ulrich, D. (1995). Tic tac test ready. *Nurse Educator, 20,* 4–7.

Glendon, K., & Ulrich, D. (1997). Unfolding cases: An experiential learning model. *Nurse Educator, 22,* 15–18.

Glendon, K., & Ulrich, D. (2001). *Unfolding case studies: Experiencing the realities of clinical nursing practice.* Upper Saddle River, NJ: Prentice-Hall.

Goodsell, A., Maber, M., & Tinto, V. (1992). *Collaborative learning: A sourcebook for higher education.* National Center on Post Secondary Teaching, Learning, and Assessment. Pennsylvania State University.

Ham, K., & O'Rourke, E. (2004). Clinical preparation for beginning nursing students: An experiential learning activity. *Nurse Educator, 29*(4), 139–141.

Hummel, F., & Peters, D. (1994). Bafa Bafa: A cultural awareness game. *Nurse Educator, 19,* 8.

Ibarreta, G., & McLeod, L. (2004). Thinking aloud on paper:An experience in journal writing. *Journal of Nursing Education, 43*(3), 134–137.

Ishikawa, K. (1982). *Guide to quality control.* White Plains, NY: Asian Productivity Organization, Kraus International Publications.

Johnson, B. (1996). *Island maps.* Proceedings of International Society for Exploring Teaching Alternative Conference. Columbus, OH.

Johnson, D., & Johnson, R. (1984). *Circles of learning: Cooperation in the classroom.* Alexandria, VA: Association for Supervision and Curriculum Development.

Johnson, D., & Johnson, R. (1989). *Cooperation and competition: Theory and research.* Edena, MN: Interaction Book Co.

Johnson, D., & Johnson, R. (1993, spring). What we know about cooperative learning at the college level. *Cooperative Learning: The Magazine for Cooperation in Higher Education, 13,* 17–18.

Johnson, D., Johnson, F., & Smith, K. (1991). *Active learning. Cooperation in the college classroom.* Edina, MN: Interaction Book Company.

Johnson, D., Johnson, F., & Smith, K. (1998). *Active learning: Cooperation in the college classroom.* Edina, MN: Interaction Book Co.

Kagan, S. (1989/1990). The structural approach to cooperative learning. *Educational Leadership, 47,* 12–15.

Kagan, S. (1992). *Cooperative learning.* San Juan Capistrano, CA: Resources for Teachers.

Kolb, D. A. (1976). *Learning styles inventory technical manual.* Boston: McBer.

Kuhn, D. (2000). Why development does (and doesn't) occur: Evidence from the domain of inductive reasoning. In R. Siegler & J. McClelland (Eds.), *Mechanisms of cognitive development: Neural & behavioral perspectives.* Mahwah, NJ: Erlbaum.

Ledlow, S. (1999). *Cooperative learning in higher education.* Center for learning and teaching excellence: Arizona State University. http://clte.asu.edu/active/mainart.htm

Lenaghan, N. (1996). Respiratory crossword puzzle. *Nurse Educator, 21,* 7–8, 14.

Locke, J. (1693). *Some thoughts concerning education.* http://www.socsci.kun.nl/ped/whp/histeduc/locke/

Lyman, F. (1987). Think-pair-share: An expanding teaching technique. *MAA-CIE Cooperative News, 1,* 1–2.

McKeachie, W. (1978). *Teaching tips: A guidebook for the beginning college teacher.* Lexington, MA: D. C. Heath & Co.

Meyers, C. (1991). *Teaching students to think critically.* San Francisco: Jossey-Bass.

Millis, B., & Cottell, P. (1998). *Cooperative learning for higher education faculty.* Phoenix, AZ: Oryz.

Mueller, A., Johnston, M., & Bligh, D. (2001). Mind-mapped careplans: A remarkable alternative to traditional nursing care plans. *Nurse Educator, 26*(2), 75–80.

Myers, I., & McCaulley, M. (1985). *Manual, a guide to the development and use of the Myers-Briggs type indicator.* Palo Alto, CA: Consulting Psychologists Press.

Parker, F., & Faulk, D. (2004). Lights, camera, action: Using feature films to stimulate emancipatory learning in the RN to BSN student. *Nurse Educator, 29*(4), 144–146.

Paul, R. (1992). *Critical thinking: What every person needs to survive in a rapidly changing world.* Santa Rosa, CA: The Foundation For Critical Thinking.

Paul, R. (1993). *Critical thinking: How to prepare students for a rapidly changing world.* Santa Rosa, CA: Foundation for Critical Thinking.

Paul, R., & Elder, L. (2001). *Critical thinking: Tools for taking charge of your learning and your life.* Upper Saddle River, NJ: Prentice Hall.

Perry, W. G. (1970). *Forms of intellectual and ethical development in the college years.* New York: Holt, Rinehart & Winston.

Qin, Z., Johnson, D., & Johnson, R. (1995). Cooperative versus competitive efforts and problem solving. *Review of Educational Research, 65,* 129–143.

Schuster, P. (2002). *Concept mapping: A critical thinking approach to care planning.* Philadelphia: F. A. Davis.

Sharan, S. (1980). Cooperative learning in small groups: Recent methods and effects on achievement, attitudes, and ethnic relations. *Review of Educational Research, 50,* 241–271.

Silberman, M. (1996). *Active learning: 101 strategies to teach any subject.* Boston: Allyn & Bacon.

Slavin, R. E. (1980). Cooperative learning. *Review of Educational Research, 50,* 315–342.

Slavin, R. E. (1983a). *Cooperative learning.* New York: Longman.

Slavin, R. E. (1983b). When does cooperative learning increase student achievement? *Psychological Bulletin, 94,* 429–445.

Solomon, R., Davidson, N., & Solomon, E. (1993). *The handbook for the fourth R: Relationship activities for cooperative and collegial learning.* Columbia, MD: National Institute for Relationship Training.

Spunt, D., Foster, D., & Adams, K. (2004). Mock code: A clinical simulation module. *Nurse Educator, 29*(5), 192–194.

Trauch, P. (2003). Student drawing: A clinical learning tool. *Nurse Educator,* *28*(2), 58–60.

Ulrich, D., & Glendon, K. (1994). Fishbone strategy: A TQM strategy applied to nursing education. *Nurse Educator, 19,* 7–8.

Ulrich, D., & Glendon, K. (1995). Jigsaw: A critical thinking experience. *Nurse Educator, 20,* 6–7.

Ulrich, D., & Glendon, K. (1997). Let's play nurse. *Nurse Educator, 22,* 9–10.

Ulrich, D., Teets, J., & Quinn, C. (1994). Using video families to teach family functioning. *Journal of Nursing Education, 33,* 1–3.

Watson, G., & Glaser, E. M. (1964). *Critical thinking appraisal.* Orlando, FL: Harcourt Brace Jovanovich.

Wong, D. (1999). *Whaley & Wong's nursing care of children* (6th ed.). St. Louis: Mosby.

Index

Springer Publishing Company

Educating Nurses for Leadership

Harriet R. Feldman, PhD, RN, FAAN
Martha J. Greenberg, PhD, RN, Editors

This book provides tools for nurse educators and administrators to prepare nurses to be effective leaders so that they may advance health care practice and the profession of nursing. Part I describes a Leadership Education Model and its six modules of leader as achiever, communicator, critical thinker, expert, mentor, and visionary. Part II presents proven strategies from schools across the United States for integrating leadership into the nursing curriculum. Part III discusses strategies that can be used in the clinical setting by administrators and staff developers. The annotated bibliography at the back of the book offers important additional resources on leadership development in nursing.

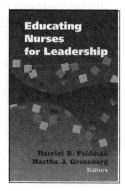

Partial Contents:

Part I: A Model for Educating Future Leaders • Preparing Nurse Leaders: A Leadership Education Model, *J.A. Lemire* • Leader as Visionary, *J. Aroian* • Leader as Expert, *B. Frank* • Leader as Achiever, *J. Dienemann* • Leader as Critical Thinker, *J.A. Lemire* • Leader as Communicator, *P.A. Haynor* • Leader as Mentor, *C. Vance*

Part II: Using Nursing History to Educate for Leadership, *S.B. Lewenson* • Reflective Journaling: Bridging the Theory-Practice Gap, *D. Morgan, J. Johnson,* and *D. Garrison* • Using Group Process to Develop Caring Leaders, *L. Wagner* • Using Parse's Theory to Educate for Leadership, *S. Ramey* and *S. Bunkers* • Educating Future Leaders Using Problem-Based Learning, *B. Williams* • Using Online Clinical Scenarios to Build Leadership Skills, *C. Wilson*

Part III: Leadership Education in the Clinical Setting • Practice-Oriented Leadership Education, *J. Aroian* and *J. Dienemann* • Using Shift Coordinators to Teach Leadership Skills Needed for NCLEX-RN, *J. Aucoin* and *S. Letvak* • Teaching the Value of Evidence-Based Practice, *B. Frank* • Developing Evidence-Based Practice Skills Through Experiential Learning, *K. Sackett* and *J. Jones* • Succession Planning as a Strategy to Prepare Future Leaders, *H. Green*

2004   352pp   hardcover   0-8261-2664-2

11 West 42nd Street, New York, NY 10036-8002 • Fax: 212-941-7842
Order Toll-Free: 877-687-7476 • Order On-line: www.springerpub.com